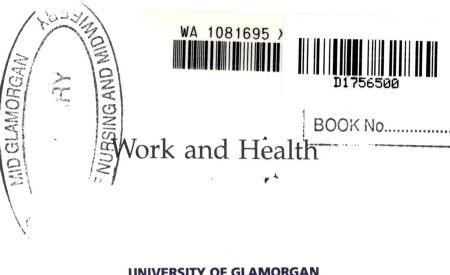

Work and Health

**UNIVERSITY OF GLAMORGAN
LEARNING RESOURCES CENTRE**

Pontypridd, Mid Glamorgan, CF37 1DL
Telephone: Pontypridd (0443) 480480

Books are to be returned on or before the last date below

For my husband, Peter

Work and Health

An introduction to occupational health care

Edited by Margaret Bamford
Director of Nursing Services
(Acting),
West Midlands Regional Health
Authority, UK

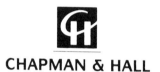

CHAPMAN & HALL

London · Glasgow · Weinheim · New York · Tokyo · Melbourne · Madras

Published by Chapman & Hall, 2–6 Boundary Row, London SE1 8HN, UK

Chapman & Hall, 2–6 Boundary Row, London SE1 8HN, UK

Blackie Academic & Professional, Wester Cleddens Road, Bishopbriggs, Glasgow G64 2NZ, UK

Chapman & Hall GmbH, Pappelallee 3, 69469 Weinheim, Germany

Chapman & Hall USA, One Penn Plaza, 41st Floor, New York NY 10119, USA

Chapman & Hall Japan, ITP-Japan, Kyowa Building, 3F, 2-2-1 Hirakawacho, Chiyoda-ku, Tokyo 102, Japan

Chapman & Hall Australia, Thomas Nelson Australia, 102 Dodds Street, South Melbourne, Victoria 3205, Australia

Chapman & Hall India, R. Seshadri, 32 Second Main Road, CIT East, Madras 600 035, India

Distributed in the USA and Canada by Singular Publishing Group Inc., 4284 41st Street, San Diego, California 92105

First edition 1995

© 1995 Chapman & Hall

Phototypeset in 10/12pt Palatino by Intype, London
Printed in Great Britain by Page Bros., Norwich

ISBN 0 412 48430 7   1 56593 199 8 (USA)

A catalogue record for this book is available from the British Library

Library of Congress Catalog Card Number: 94–68777

∞ Printed on permanent acid-free text paper, manufactured in accordance with ANSI/NISO Z39.48–1992 and ANSI/NISO Z39.48–1984 (Permanence of Paper).

Contents

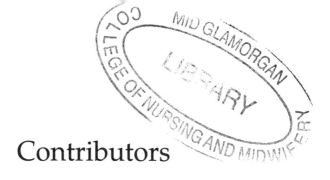

Contributors

Cynthia Atwell
Principal OHN Adviser, British Rail

Dr Margaret Bamford
Director of Nursing (Acting), West Midlands Regional Health Authority, UK

Dr Frederick Barwell
Consultant Psychologist and Honorary Research Fellow, Health Services Management Centre, University of Birmingham, UK

Andrew Cameron
Senior Lecturer, University of Wolverhampton, UK

Ann Foster
Senior Employment Nursing Adviser, Health and Safety Executive, Department of Employment, London, UK

Jane Molloy
Lecturer in Health Promotion, Institute of Advance Nursing Education, Royal College of Nursing, London, UK

Prof. Peter Spurgeon
Director of Research and Consultancy, Health Services Management Centre, University of Birmingham, UK

Michael Whincup
Senior Lecturer in Law, Barrister, University of Keele, UK

1

Introduction to occupational health

Margaret Bamford

This book is about the interaction between health and work. It is intended to provide a framework for health professionals to consider when they are working with people, and caring for them, in the community, in hospital, in general practice, at work, or in any setting where an understanding of the effects of work on health and health on work would be to the benefit of the patient or client.

Occupational health (OH), or work health, has been documented for many years. We have known since antiquity that work can damage a person: that is why the Greeks and Romans made slaves and criminals do the hazardous work in mines and quarries. In those early times no association was made between work and health. In the mid–1500s two writers described the hazards of mining, not in relation to health but rather as a social commentary or justification: Agricola (1493–1555) and Paracelsus (1493–1541). Agricola found that:

> in the mines of the Carpathian mountains, women are found who have married seven husbands, all of whom this terrible consumption has carried off to a premature death.
>
> (Schilling, 1973, p. 4)

He advocated the use of veils across the face to protect the miners from whatever it was that was giving them consumption. Paracelsus has a different view on the topic. He felt that:

> We must have gold and silver, also other metals, iron, tin,

copper, lead and mercury. If we wish to have these, we must risk both life and body in a struggle with many enemies that oppose us.

(Schilling, 1973, p. 4)

By the use of the term enemies he could have meant the environment, or indeed people who were voicing their concerns about the loss of life associated with obtaining these metals.

Other writers have described the 'evils of work'. One was Bernardino Ramazzini (1633–1714), a physician and Professor of Medicine in Modena and Padua, in Italy. His book, published in 1700, described the diseases of occupations as he observed them in Modena. He advocated that doctors should visit the town's workshops and observe the activities of the people who did the work which supported the community. He also suggested that:

'When you come to a patient's house, you should ask him what sort of pains he has, what caused them, how many days has he been ill, whether the bowels are working and what sort of food he eats.' So says Hippocrates in his work Affections. I may venture to add one more question: What occupation does he follow?

(Ramazzini, 1700 [trans. W. C. Wright, 1964, p. 13])

Elizabeth Gaskell (1810–1865) was an eminent Victorian author who wrote *The Life of Charlotte Bronte* (Gaskell, 1975). She also wrote novels about her time such as *North and South* (Gaskell, 1970), which described the activities and realities of them, graphically describing some of the occupational health conditions that prevailed:

'Fluff,' repeated Bessy, 'Little bits as fly off fro' the cotton, when they're carding it, and fill the air till it looks all fine white dust. They say it winds around the lungs, and tightens them up. Anyhow, there's many a one as works in a carding-room, that falls into a waste, coughing and spitting blood, because they're just poisoned by the fluff.'

(Gaskell, 1970, p. 146)

Occupational ill health and disease were known to occurr, but nobody had the knowledge and skill to prevent it. Accidents and disease in the workplace were seen as part and parcel of every-day life, bad luck, carelessness, no one's fault, particularly not the owners. Some changes were affected in working conditions in the early 1800s. These changes primarily affected the working conditions of children, then gradually extended to include women, and finally to cover men's working conditions (Southgate, 1965; Schilling, 1973).

Sir Thomas Legge (1863–1932) was the first Medical Inspector of Factories in 1898. When he resigned from the inspectorate in 1926 because the then government would not ratify an international convention prohibiting the use of white lead for the inside painting of buildings, he became the Medical Advisor to the TUC (Lloyd Davies, 1957). He had views on issues in the workplace which were ahead of his time. He said:

> unless and until the employer has done everything – and everything means a good deal – the workman can do next to nothing to protect himself, although he is naturally willing enough to do his share.
>
> (Legge, 1934, p. 3)

So there was a move to say that people at work needed more protection than had previously been provided. This was seen in the development of legislation which placed major responsibilities on employers, and some responsibilities on employed persons. However, problems still occurred, and are still occurring. Lloyd Davies (1957, p. 6) put the problem into perspective for most people in society:

> A workman's capital is his health and his ability to work; without these assets he is bankrupt.

It is in no one's interest to have a population damaged by work. The difficulty is for some decision-makers to decide what proportion of a population a community can afford to have damaged, and still be viable. This is an aspect of risk management and society has always had an element of that thinking in its make-up.

Until the beginning of this century, little or no attention was paid to the effects of work on health. Certain facts came to light because of other events: the male population was not strong enough to be a proper army to fight the Boers during the late 1800s and again in the First World War. This made people look at all aspects of social conditions: work, housing, diet, health, medicine, sanitation. The subsequent depression in the

1920–1930s made major progress in health-related issues difficult to achieve. The greatest achievements arose out of the efforts put into the Second World War. The rapid growth in technology arising out of this event have not been paralleled at any other time in history; with it came the technology, knowledge and skills to do something about workplace hazards.

Workplace health developed outside the arrangements for health in the community as a whole. It was seen as something separate and distinct and needed to be dealt with in a different way. Occupational health and safety became the responsibility of the various government departments that dealt with employment issues, the Ministry of Labour and the Department of Employment, rather than the Department of Health. This has meant that many health professionals do not have an understanding of the effects of work on health, and are therefore in some circumstances ignorant of the other possible factors that need to be taken into account when caring for people and their health needs in a community.

If you would like to read more about the history of occupational health there is a small reading list given at the end of this chapter. Some of these references will seem old to today's younger readers, but they are easy to read and would make a good start before you move on to more modern writers.

WHAT IS UNDERSTOOD BY THE TERM OCCUPATIONAL HEALTH?

There is an international definition of occupational health which it would probably be helpful to consider. The World Health Organisation (WHO) have produced this definition:

1. To identify and bring under control at the workplace all chemical, physical, mechanical, biological and psychosocial agents that are known to be or suspected of being hazardous;
2. to ensure that the physical and mental demands imposed on people at work by their respective jobs are properly matched with their individual, anatomical, physiological and psychological capabilities, needs and limitations;
3. to provide effective measures to protect those who are especially vulnerable to adverse working conditions.

(WHO, 1975)

This is looking at the person in the round in relation to the work they do, people who are strong or vulnerable, people who are exposed to substances or work processes. It means trying to make sure that work does the person no harm. These factors need to be considered in relation to the wider concepts underpinning health.

HEALTH FOR ALL BY THE YEAR 2000

In 1985, the WHO Regional Office for Europe published *Targets for Health for All* (WHO, 1985). This publication arose out of the Alma Ata conference 1978, and Health for all by the Year 2000. The European targets have three main foci: the promotion of lifestyles conducive to health, the reduction of preventable conditions, and the provision of care which is adequate, accessible and acceptable to all (WHO, 1985).

There is a particular target which relates to the working environment: target 25:

> By 1995, people of the region should be effectively protected against work related health risks. The achievement of this target will require the introduction of appropriate occupational health services to cover the needs of all workers;
>
> the development of health criteria for the protection of workers against biological, chemical and physical hazards;
>
> the implementation of technical and educational measures to reduce work related risk factors;
>
> and the safeguarding of specially vulnerable groups of workers.
>
> (WHO, 1985, p. 92)

This target, while addressing health in the workplace, is in reality putting workplace health into the broader perspective of health in its totality. By including workplace health in these targets for health the concept that health in the workplace should not be a separate issue is emphasized. All aspects of a person's health and well-being should be addressed, not parts of that health put into various boxes and only addressed by some individuals. There is the suggestion that in order to meet these targets, Occupational Health Services (OHS) need to meet the health needs of people who work in their own homes. In the UK, it would be an achievement if we met the health needs of people who are in formal workplaces.

> *Think about some of the people you have had to care for. What work did they do? What health or ill health condition did they have that you were offering them care for? Was there any relationship with their work? Could they explain what work they did? Could you understand what they were describing?*

OCCUPATIONAL HEALTH SERVICES

Occupational health services are provided on a voluntary basis by employers to meet the health needs of people at work. In the UK up to half the workforce has little or no regular access to an occupational health service. The provision of occupational health services is usually in larger organizations; people in small organizations have little or no access to occupational health advice (HSE, 1985). This means that when an employed person is ill or requires health advice in relation to his working conditions, the average health professional will be unable to help with specific problems. This is because they do not have specific knowledge of the underlying principles of occupational health and in many organizations there will not be a health professional to whom they can refer.

In a House of Lords select committee enquiry into the provision of occupational health services, headed by Lord Gregson (House of Lords, 1983), one of the main conclusions was that General Practitioners (GP) should take a greater interest in occupational health and be in the forefront of providing support for workplace health issues in their community. There has not been an overwhelming rush for this area of work to be developed as a legitimate area of primary care. However, the Health and Safety Executive (HSE) has recently published a booklet, *Your Patients and their Work,* which is an introduction to occupational health for family doctors (HSE, 1992), and a smaller leaflet, *What your doctor needs to know: your work and your health* (HSE, 1992). This should help in moving towards a shared understanding of the work-health interaction.

The International Labour Organisation (ILO) gave a definition of occupational health services in its Convention 161:

Occupational health services means services entrusted with essentially preventive functions and responsibilities for advising the employer, the workers and their representatives in the undertaking on:

(i) the requirements for establishing and maintaining a safe and healthy working environment which will facilitate optimal physical and mental health in relation to work;

(ii) the adaptation of work to the capabilities of workers in the light of their state of physical and mental health.

(HSC, 1986, p. 4)

The UK was a signatory to this convention, and was therefore an active player in defining what was meant in the definition. Some additional work undertaken by a group of WHO representatives looked at the issue of occupational health as a component of primary care. In the UK, OH is not seen as a part of primary care. This group, who had the advantage of being able to bring their collective expertise to this issue, described the various ways in which workers' health could be organized:

1. Community or private primary health care services provide diagnosis and treatment for general ill health; community-based occupational health units (governmental, supported by trade unions or voluntary funds or social security funds, or commercial) provide preventive OH services (environmental and medical).

2. Community-based primary health services provide care for general ill health; the medical part of preventive OH service (preventive health examinations) is provided by community-based OH units, while the environmental part is work-place-based.

3. Community-based primary health service provide care for general ill-health, while complete preventive OH activities (both environmental and medical) are workplace-based.

4. Total workers' health service (primary health care component and entire preventive OH component) is workplace-based.

(WHO, 1986, p. 9)

The model most frequently used in the UK would be number 3, a division of labour between two different services.

The development of OHS in the UK has been fragmented and piecemeal. There is no legal requirement placed on employers, and therefore some employers do not provide any service other than the minimum requirement to have a first-aider, and first-aid provision (HSE, 1981). The type of OHS provided in various workplaces are as many and different as there are industries. Some organizations provide a comprehensive **treatment service**. Others provide no treatment service at all apart from the statutory **first-aid service**. Some organizations which use hazardous or toxic substances have sophisticated **medical services** which offer **screening programmes** as well as sophisticated medical interventions to individuals. The screening programmes start before the person is even taken into employment, and are carried on throughout working life until retirement. This is part of **health supervision**. Some employees are offered a continuing screening programme even after they have left the organization or retired. Examples of this would be in the rubber industry where people have been exposed to beta-naphthylamine in the manufacture of rubber tyres, and people in other workplaces who have been exposed to dusts which could cause pneumoconiosis.

Some organizations offer comprehensive **health education** or **health promotion** programmes which take on not only the potential hazards associated with the workplace, but also lifestyle health issues such as smoking and alcohol abuse. Many organizations are very concerned with **safety issues**, and in some the occupational health service should really be called the occupational safety service, because all the energy goes into accident prevention rather than a balanced approach towards health and safety. Another aspect of occupational health service which has been a major development of the late twentieth century has been the emerging science of **occupational hygiene**. This involves taking scientific readings of the atmosphere in the workplace, monitoring the contaminants present, and also monitoring and evaluating the preventive measures in place to prevent people being exposed to the contaminants. In some cases the only protection that can be offered is the wearing of **protective clothing** or **equipment**; in other cases there are complicated exhaust ventilation systems, or other **environmentally controlled** systems which regulate processes and exposure to substances. In others there are sophisticated **remote control mechanisms** which distance the worker from a process or the substances used.

In other organizations there has developed a comprehensive **rehabilitation** service. In some instances this development was a result of the trauma and injury caused by working conditions, such as workplace accidents. Some organizations are now using these developed services to support people returning to work following other health incidents such as coronary heart disease or new diagnosis of conditions such as diabetes, asthma and epilepsy. The groundwork of the rehabilitation part of the OHS arose out of the lack of national provision before the Second World War, and the need to maintain production and effort during and following the war when the manufacturing base was so important for the nation's economy, and people were urgently needed to return to work.

Think about occupational health services you have come into contact with. Ask other people you know if they have any experience of occupational health services. What type of service was it? What was the range of services offered? Who were the personnel involved?

SHARED RESPONSIBILITY IN OCCUPATIONAL HEALTH

The various workers' associations have had a long and strong involvement in health and safety in the workplace. Most of the early pioneering work was done in partnership with the employer and the trade unions. In the early days of industrial development the energy of the trade unions and friendly societies moved the issues forward, and brought about change and development in the workplace. By law the ultimate responsibility for health and safety is the employer's, but trade unions see themselves as having a major role to play in the partnership between employer, employee and trade organization.

The European Community is now beginning to influence what happens in all member states. An example of this in the UK was the implementation of the *Control of Substances Hazardous to Health Regulations 1988* (COSHH) (HMSO, 1988). There was a specific need to provide protection at work for people exposed to substances which had the potential for being hazardous to health. The COSHH regulations are a major legislative event in occupational health care. They demonstrate a change in thinking in that the person is looked at in the round as far as work is concerned and in relation to all employment. These regulations acknowledge that occupational disease is as important as occupational accidents; they provide a systematic framework for the analysis of the interaction between exposure to substances by individuals and the control mechanisms instituted in the workplace to prevent exposure to substances. The employer has a duty to analyse substances used in the workplace, to make an assessment of risk associated with that substance, to keep a live database which will allow him to manage appropriate control mechanisms, and prevent the occurrence of occupational disease. Each person who is working with substances which are hazardous to health will have a record card detailing the substance and their exposure. Some people who are exposed to specified substances will have to undergo **medical surveillance**: this will be special medical examinations at specified times.

All health-care providers should ask people they are caring for who they know are working if they come under the COSHH regulations at work. If the answer is yes, then the health practitioner knows there are potentially specific considerations to be made.

A major cause for concern among occupational health professionals is the lack of real understanding of the total number of people who are affected by occupational disease. One of the main problems in this area of work is the long latent development period often associated with occupational disease. Today, with the problems of getting and keeping work, this can cover an employment career which may span many employers. Hashemi (1989) tried to put costs to the problem of occupational disease; he feels that far more people are killed by occupational disease than by occupational accidents. Harrington and Seaton (1988) feel there is an under-recording of the true incidence of occupational disease in the UK by a factor of two or three. There is a need to do more work in this area. The HSC recently commissioned a 'special health and safety supplement to the 1990 Labour Force Survey conducted by the Office of Population, Censuses and Surveys' (HSC, 1991). This survey, which covered some 40,000 households and nearly 80,000 respondents living in England and Wales, found the following:

an annual total of just under 1.5 million work related injuries, of which rather more than half a million came within the RIDDOR definition;

something over 2 million people suffering from illness which they believe to have been caused or made worse by their work;

work-related injuries and ill health giving rise to around 29 million days off work a year – equivalent to just over one day for every worker.

(HSC, 1991, p. 55)

RIDDOR is the Reporting of Injuries, Diseases and Dangerous Occurrences Regulations 1985, and sets the framework for what must be reported nationally. HSE will be doing further work in this area, but it is important to understand that some people do not know what to report and some people deliberately withhold information. Either way, it is a problem for planners and providers of service if the true picture does not emerge.

OCCUPATIONAL ACCIDENTS

There is still concern about the number of fatal accidents which are occurring in the workplace. The 1990–91 annual report of the Health and Safety Commission (HSC, 1991), which is the policy arm of the Department of Employment's Health and Safety Executive (HSE), had the following statement in the chairman's foreword:

the picture in other sectors has shown no improvement from the levels which the Commission has consistently emphasised are unacceptably high. Fatalities to employees appear to have levelled off at about 360 in recent years.

(HSC, 1991, pp. ix–x)

There is concern for the issue of accidents in the workplace, for many of them could be avoided. We know how many fatal accidents there are in all sectors of industry each year – 538 in 1991 – and how many people suffer major injuries – 30,684 (HSC, 1991). However, we do not know how many people suffer from minor injuries. These must be considerable and they have the potential to go on and cause personal discomfort, pain and possibly further complications. Minor injuries may not be recorded and may not receive appropriate treatment and care.

In 1981–82 there were 7,000,000 new spells of certified incapacity for sickness due to prescribed diseases and industrial injuries, and in the late 1980s there was a steady figure of 145,000 people receiving Industrial Disablement Benefit (Webb and Schilling, 1988). Perhaps now with the recession there may be changes to these numbers, but the issue is still about in society, and the health service has to deal with the end product of these issues.

THE HEALTH OF THE NATION

The first government green paper on *The Health of the Nation* (HMSO, 1991) gave scant consideration to the workplace as a place where health initiatives could take place or preventive activities were appropriate. William Waldegrave who was then Secretary of State for Health identified three main points in his foreword: first, that the document was about the prevention of ill health and the promotion of good health; second, that there was a need for people to change their behaviour; and third that the setting of objectives and targets would provide a disciplined approach towards improving health (HMSO, 1991). This document identified major challenges that need to be addressed in our communities:

- to increase understanding of the state of the population's health and what influences it;

- to reduce exposure to risks from people's own behaviour or the environment which damages health;

- to take action to ensure that people are properly informed and have the freedom to exercise choice. People cannot be forced to behave sensibly in terms of their smoking, eating, exercise, alcohol or sexual habits;

- to continue to improve the efficiency, effectiveness and quality of NHS care; and

- for government or others, to take effective action on behalf of the community as a whole, to monitor and, when necessary, to eliminate or minimise the threats to individuals from the external world which they cannot themselves control.

(HMSO, 1991, pp. viii-ix)

Readers could have been excused for thinking that this statement would have included the workplace as a focal point for many of the ideas expressed in these statements. Even now it is difficult for the Department of Health to affect major change and initiatives in the workplace: there is still not the integration of knowledge and understanding of workplace health and safety issues into mainstream health provision. Yet many of the challenges listed above could have sensibly been targeted at the workplace, and could have seen some changes made to the health of people at work. It is important to remember that these people earn the wealth which allows the country to buy its goods and services, which make it possible to provide services such as the health service for the rest of the community.

THE HEALTH OF THE NATION APPLIED TO THE WORKPLACE

The Health of the Nation targets are clear and objective. They are:

Coronary heart disease and stroke

- To reduce the death rate for both CHD and stroke in people under 65 by at least 40% by the year 2000.
- To reduce the death rate for CHD in people aged 65 to 74 by at least 30% by the year 2000.
- To reduce the death rate for stroke in people aged 65 to 74 by at least 40% by the year 2000.

Cancers

- To reduce the death rate for breast cancer in the population invited for screening by at least 25% by the year 2000.
- To reduce the incidence of invasive cervical cancer by at least 20% by the year 2000.
- To halt the year-on-year increase in the incidence of skin cancer by 2005.
- To reduce the death rate for lung cancer by at least 30% in men under 75 and 15% in women under 75 by 2010.

Mental illness

- To improve significantly the health and social functioning of mentally ill people. To reduce the overall suicide rate by at least 15% by the year 2000.
- To reduce the suicide rate of severely mentally ill people by at least 33% by the year 2000.

HIV/AIDS and sexual health

- To reduce the incidence of gonorrhoea among men and women aged 15–64 by at least 20% by 1995.
- To reduce the percentage of injecting drug users who report sharing injecting equipment in the previous four weeks by at least 50% by 1997, and by at least a further 50% by the year 2000.
- To reduce the rate of conceptions among the under–16s by at least 50% by the year 2000.

Accidents

- To reduce the death rate for accidents among children aged under 15 by at least 33% by 2005.
- To reduce the death rate for accidents among young people aged 15 to 24 by at least 25% by 2005.
- To reduce the death rate for accidents among people aged 65 and over by at least 33% by 2005 (HMSO, 1992).

All these targets could be focused on the workplace. There would be a captive audience of men and women who could be influenced by health promotion and educational activities.

In some industries there could be a very specific action which would target exposure to substances thought to cause ill health, such as the study of exposure of viscose-rayon workers to carbon-disulphide in Finland (Sweetman, Taylor and Elwood, 1987). The study showed that those exposed workers were five times more likely to die of heart disease than non-exposed workers. In other workplaces attention to the provision of nutritionally sound food and snacks and access to exercise facilities would be positive ways of helping people in the community work towards reducing heart disease.

Some cancers are occupationally induced: asbestos workers, rubber workers, people who are exposed to bright sunshine for long periods are all vulnerable. The control and containment of substances and activities in the workplace could contribute to achieving these overall targets.

Mental illness has many causes: who knows what would be the final trigger that pushed a person out of their equilibrium and into mental illness? It could be that occupational stress is the cause: poor working conditions, inflexible working hours, authoritarian management styles, or production methods which are machine driven, such as assembly lines. A consideration of workplace activities by such people as members of the primary health care team could help those who are in crisis.

The whole area of HIV/AIDS has implications for the health care industry, the law enforcement services and the prison service. These people are at the forefront of exposure by virtue of their occupational roles. Although accidental exposure and contamination is not a major threat to these occupational groups, they, through their roles, have an opportunity to educate others and demonstrate 'good practice'. This good practice could relate to the wearing of protective clothing when handling any blood products, disposing of equipment efficiently and effectively, and communication of the process to the person they are dealing with together with a rationale for their actions.

A reduction of accidents in any society is to be welcomed. It would seem from the published targets that the reduction of accidents in the 25–64-year age groups is not to be a priority for the NHS; this can only mean that it remains a responsibility of the Department of Employment. This could mean that the NHS will be able to ignore this age group when producing policy, defining contracts for health care or assessing the needs of a community.

THE NHS AS A HEALTHY EMPLOYER

The recent *The Health of the Nation* (HMSO, 1992) raised the issue of healthy work places and placed an obligation on the NHS not only to address this issue internally but to be a lead agent in establishing partnerships with other employers to move them to producing a healthy workplace. Many of the larger organizations will have occupational health services which are far more pro-active and sophisticated than the occupational services in the NHS, which does put the NHS at a disadvantage in this exercise. The lead agency nationally for this activity is the Health Education Authority (HEA).

The main thrust of these activities applied to the NHS is through a 12-point programme:

1. Raise awareness of health at work and healthy living;
2. Production of a smoking policy, to provide smoking venues, stop sales of tobacco on NHS premises;

3. Provide and promote healthy choices for food;
4. Promote sensible drinking, and provide support for problem drinkers;
5. Introduce physical activity programmes;
6. Promote positive mental health;
7. Encourage positive attitudes to sex;
8. Provide opportunities for all staff to have health checks and attend screenings, and appropriate follow-ups;
9. Explore changes that can be made within the work situation (this relates to environmental issues, not ergonomic issues);
10. Review health, hygiene and safety practices;
11. Develop management practices and monitoring systems;
12. Design a training strategy to support health initiatives and reinforce health-promoting behaviour.

(HEA/NHSME, 1992)

While acknowledging that there needs to be a national activity in relation to workplace health, it is disappointing that this initiative does not go further and is not managed in conjunction with the HSE. This means that health professionals who have little or no experience of the workplace will be attempting to make new relationships with organizations with whom they will have had no previous experience. This will result in energy being put into activities which could be short-circuited by using HSE colleagues.

PROFESSIONALS IN OCCUPATIONAL HEALTH

There are a range of people who are involved in occupational health delivery. These range from first-aiders to scientists, but the mainstay of many services are the occupational health nurse and doctor. Occupational health teams tend to be employed in the larger organizations which themselves are more sophisticated and structured as organizations than small businesses and firms (HSC, 1977). This means that all people who work do not have access to an occupational health service. These teams usually consist of occupational health nurses and doctors, together with safety personnel, occupational hygienists, ergonomists and physiotherapists. Some organizations employ counsellors who address individual's concerns which are personal to them, but which can affect their work. Additional information on the range of professionals involved, and the educational and training requirements and opportunities available, can be found in a booklet produced by the co-ordinating committee of the professional occupational health and safety organizations (POHSO, 1986).

THE FUTURE

What does the future hold for people who work in the UK? Work is changing. Job opportunities in the traditional sense are not available. What do people do? What does the government do? Does it make a concerted effort to make work for people at any cost, or does it decide that there will be certain people who will never work and support them by state subsidy? How long can that be afforded? People are brought up to think that work is something which is done after leaving school, but it may not be work in the way we have always thought it was.

What is to be done about the health of people who work? If fewer people are working to produce the wealth to support the social infrastructure of the country, should we look after those people better? Should we have positive discrimination in their favour as far as health care is concerned?

WHAT DO PEOPLE WHO WORK THINK ABOUT THEIR HEALTH?

In a recent study of people who were at work (Bamford, 1993), which asked people at work if they thought they were healthy, 92% felt that they were. This was a study of fourteen different organizations in the West Midlands; 960 questionnaires were sent out and 459 were returned: a 48% response rate. The sample was divided into senior managers, middle managers and operatives. When asked to consider if their health was above average, average or below average compared to someone of a similar age, 34% felt that they were above average, 58% felt that they were average and 7% felt that their health was below average. In other research done, but of whole populations rather than specifically targeted ones like the people at work, the results are slightly different. Hanney (1979) looked at a population in Glasgow; 27% of those people felt that their health was perfect, 65% felt their health was good or fair and 7% felt that their health was poor or very poor. This last figure is the same as for the people at work. However, the people in Bamford's group are at work; the people in Hanney's group may or may not be at work: they may be the chronic sick people in a community.

The people in Bamford's (1993) study also have clear perceptions about factors which have an effect on their health. The effects of work on health was seen as having a more negative effect; lifestyle on health was seen as having a more positive effect and the effects of leisure on health were also seen as having a positive effect. People at work are able to describe how they feel, what things are important to them, how they manage their health, what services they use, when they use them and what for. Health professionals need to tap into this tremendous wealth of experience and use it for their own education and to assist them in understanding and caring for people in the community.

ABOUT THIS BOOK

This book will not cover all the issues in relation to occupational health, but it is intended to cover those issues which health professionals need to know something about, and which can give them a basis for further study and research. It is hoped that the issues covered in these subsequent chapters will give a feeling for the current and relevant issues which need to be considered and addressed by other professional groups in their caring for people who have become ill, either through occupational or non-occupational disease, and for those who need to offer people in their care support and preventive approaches to looking after their health and well-being.

Chapters Two and Three address the important areas of the effects of work on health and health on work. The symbiotic relationship between these two factors needs to be understood by health professionals in their caring relationship with people in a community.

Chapter Two, by Ann Foster, explores the major concerns in relation to the effects of work on health: manual handling; occupational lung disease and cancers. Other occupational health conditions are identified and all are considered in relation to the effect they can have on a person's health. This is a chapter which for some people will be a new concept; for others it will extend and confirm what they had already been aware of. For all readers there is hopefully something new in the chapter to extend their thinking and to benefit patient and client care.

Chapter Three, by Cynthia Atwell, looks at the other side of the equation. What do the effects of a person's health bring to their work? What effects does this health, or its absence, have on their ability to perform and function at work? What are the implications for doing particular types of work? What precautions need to be taken? How will other people be affected? What safeguards do employers need to take, and what advice do health professionals need to give to people returning to work after sickness or injury?

Chapter Four, by Andrew Cameron, addresses the important area of sociology of the workplace. The more acknowledgement there is of the social dimensions of work, the better will be the understanding of its importance in dealing with the whole person in relation to their health and their family's health. The social dynamics of the workplace give many people their place in society. They can also be the cause of much ill health and disease, and need to be taken on board by health professionals as potential causes of conflict, tension and stress in individuals.

Chapter Five, by Peter Spurgeon and Fred Barwell, addresses the relationship of the individual in relation to work and its many and various demands. So much can be done to address the health needs of people at work by considering their psychological and psychosocial needs. Consideration of the individual in the workplace is as important as the consideration of the individual in the family or community. For some people the workplace *is* their family and community.

Chapter Six, by Jane Molloy, is a chapter on the potential contribution of health professionals to the health of the employed population, through the opportunity to address health issues in a structured and realistic way. There is emphasis on caring for and educating the whole person on issues which can affect them at work, at play and at rest. The argument is made and substantiated for the use of the workplace as a focus for health promotion.

Chapter Seven, by Michael Whincup, spells out the legal framework for regulating the workplace and as such should be of personal interest to any reader who also works. He clearly describes the legal framework which must apply to, and also legal definitions which underpin action in the workplace.

Examples and interpretation is given of primary legislation and case law which will serve to illustrate the underlying issues to be addressed in understanding employment law.

FURTHER READING: HISTORY OF OCCUPATIONAL HEALTH

Charley, I.H. (1954) *The Birth of Industrial Nursing*, Bailliere Tindall and Cox, London.

Ramazzini, B. (1964) *Diseases of Workers* (trans. W.C. Wright), Hafner, New York.

Schilling, R.S.F. (1973) *Occupational Health Practice*, Butterworths, London.

Southgate, G.W. (1965) *English Economic History*, Dent, London.

REFERENCES

Bamford, M. (1993) *Aspects of Health among an Employed Population*, PhD thesis, Aston University, Birmingham.

Gaskell, E. (1970) *North and South*, Penguin Classics, London. (First published 1854–5 in *Household Works*.)

Gaskell, E. (1975) *The Life of Charlotte Bronte*, Penguin Books, London. (First published 1857.)

Hanney, D.R. (1979) *The Symptom Iceburg*, Routledge and Kegan Paul, London.

Harrington, J.M. and Seaton, A. (1988) A payroll tax for occupational health research. *British Medical Journal*, **296**, 1618.

Hashemi, K. (1989) *Hazards of the Fork Lift Truck*, MD thesis, University of Birmingham.

HSC (1977) *Occupational Health Services: The Way Ahead*, HMSO, London.

HSC (1986) *International Labour Organisation, Convention 161 and Recommendation 171 on Occupational Health Services. A Consultative Document*, HSE, HMSO, London.

HSC (1991) *Annual Report, 1990–91*, HMSO, London.

HSE (1981) *First Aid at Work*, HS(R)11, HMSO, London.

HSE (1985) *Health at Work: 1983–85. Employment Medical Advisory Service Report*, HMSO, London.

HSE (1992) *Your Patients and their work*, HMSO, London.

HSE (1992) *What your Doctor Needs to Know: your Work and your Health*, HMSO, London.

HMSO (1988) *Control of Substances Hazardous to Health Regulations 1988*, HMSO, London.

HMSO (1991) *The Health of the Nation*, HMSO, London.

HMSO (1992) *The Health of the Nation*, HMSO, London.

House of Lords (1983) *Select Committee on Science and Technology: Occupational Health and Hygiene Services*, Vol. 1, HMSO, London.

Legge, T.M. (1934) *Industrial Maladies*, (ed.) S.A. Henry, Oxford University Press, London.

Lloyd Davies, T.A. (1957) *The Practice of Industrial Medicine*, Churchill, London.

POHSO (1986) *Co-ordinating Committee for Professional Occupational Health Safety Organisations*, POHSO, University of Reading.

Ramazzini, B. (1964) *Diseases of Workers* (trans. W.C. Wright), Hafner, New York.

Schilling, R.S.F. (1973) *Occupational Health Practice*, Butterworths, London.

Sweetman, P.M., Taylor, S.W.C. and Elwood, P.C. (1987) Exposure to carbon-disulphide and ischaemic heart disease in a viscose rayon factory. *British Journal of Industrial Medicine*, **44**, 220–7.

Webb, T. and Schilling, R. (1988) *Health at Work: A Report on Health Promotion in the Workplace*. Research Report No. 22, HEA, London.

WHO (1975) *Environmental and Health Monitoring in Occupational Health*. Technical Report No. 535, WHO, Geneva.

WHO (1985) *Targets for Health for All. Targets in support of the European Regional Strategy for Health for All*, WHO, Copenhagen.

WHO (1986) *Occupational Health as a Component of Primary Health Care*, WHO, Copenhagen.

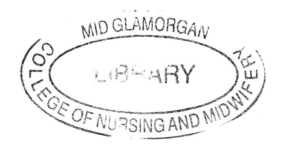

2

The effects of work on health

Ann Foster

INTRODUCTION

It is an unfortunate fact of life that most of us need to work. Some find it fulfilling and more than just financially rewarding. Others are content with their pay-packet or cheque at the end of the week or month.

I wonder how many of us reflect on the relationship between work and health and the health of our patients or clients? In accident terms it may be obvious, for example the effect of moving machinery coming into contact with our hands or fingers. Accident and Emergency Departments (A&E) have long played host to workplace-safety failures, but what about the less obvious effects of work on health?

These may range from illness directly related to occupation, such as mesothelioma in (former) asbestos workers, to ill health exacerbated by occupation, such as dermatitis exacerbated by working with skin irritants. Furthermore, the effect of work on health may not be immediate. The lapse of time (latency period) between exposure to asbestos and developing mesothelioma may be as long as 30 to 40 years. Despite some difficulty in identifying the exact amount of ill health related to work, it is possible to take guidance from statistics which show that about 5,500 people each year qualify for compensation because of work-related disease (Department of Social Security). This figure may represent only the small number of people claiming under the Social Security Act 1975 (HMSO, 1975) (see references later in this chapter). The number of people whose health is actually affected by work is much higher.

It is worth considering the questions:

1. Why should nurses and health-care workers be interested in the effects of work on health?

2. How can knowledge about the effects of work on health improve my practice?

3. Is there an occupational health service (OHS) at my patient's or client's workplace who can advise?

The provision of an on-site OHS in industry varies between the public and the private sector and by size of the undertaking (HSE, 1992d). This leaves a considerable number of the working population who may have work-related health problems without access to specialist advice. By having some knowledge about the effect of work on health, nurses and other health-care workers can widen the scope and effectiveness of their practice in caring for their patients and clients. The editor of this book has commented:

> The more people who are knowledgable doers, the more benefits will be felt in the population.
>
> (Bamford, 1992)

As an occupational health practitioner, I see all health-care workers as potential intermediaries in promoting occupational health. Thus the comment above can be paraphrased:

> The more people who are knowledgable doers, the more benefits will be found in the workplace.

Workers and the population at large are indivisible.

SOME EFFECTS OF WORK ON HEALTH

This chapter will discuss some of the immediate and some of the latent effects of work on health. It will use as the starting point the potential workplace hazard, give examples of occupations where the hazard may be present and outline some manifestations. It is not intended to provide a physiological or toxicological description of effects on individual organs or body systems. References are provided for readers who wish to pursue this.

The aim is to encourage readers to consider:

1. What work does my patient/client do? What work have they done in the past?

2. Could their problem be affected by that work?

3. If so, what can I do to help my patient/client?

Although this chapter will concentrate on illness arising out of work activity, it is worth remembering that workplace accidents have an obvious effect on health.

The largest group of accidents reported annually to the Health and Safety Executive (HSE) or to Local Authorities (LA) are those associated with manual handling: that is, the transporting or supporting of loads by hand or by bodily force. The introduction to the *Guidance on Regulations, Manual Handling Operations Regulations 1992* (HSE, 1992c) states that 34% of accidents causing injury are related to manual handling and result in over-three-day injury. These are injuries resulting in absence from normal work of more than three days which should be notified to the HSE or the LA, whichever is responsible for regulating health and safety at the particular workplace where the accident happened. The Guidance Notes state:

> Poor posture and excessive repetition of movement can be important factors in (their) onset. Many manual handling injuries are cumulative rather than being attributable to any single handling incident. A full recovery is not always made; the result can be physical impairment or even permanent disability.

> (HSE, 1992c, p. 1)

Of course, health-care workers may well be aware of this effect of work on health. During 1990 and 1991, over-three-day injuries in medical, veterinary and other health services accounted for 55% of those injuries reported. However, statistics reveal that other industries reporting between 20%–30% manual handling injuries include agricultural workers, manufacturing industries, chemical industries, mechanical and electrical engineering, motor-vehicle manufacturers and repairers, food, drink and tobacco industries, textile manufacturers, timber and furniture industries and the construction industry. These injuries are not only costly in terms of pain and discomfort to the individual sufferer but also costly to the employer and society as a whole (HSE, 1992c).

Just as it may be difficult to identify the exact time at which these types of injuries may occur, other effects of work on health may also be difficult to pinpoint. In order to encourage you to consider this dimension in relation to your patient/client, the Tables 2.1–2.5 show examples of the types of hazards commonly encountered in the workplace. These may be classified as chemical hazards, physical hazards, biological hazards, ergonomic hazards and organizational hazards. Examples of occupations where these hazards arise are identified and in the final column of the table there is a list of possible effects on health arising from that work.

The tables are not exhaustive either in possible hazard or effect on health. The intention is to alert you to situations in which your patients'/clients' ill health may be work-related.

The result of exposure to a hazard in the workplace is influenced by the type of substance and the circumstances of exposure: the length of time of exposure and the concentration of the substance.

As a result of exposure, substances may gain entry to the worker's body by any (or all) of three routes: inhalation, ingestion or skin absorption. From the examples used in the tables, substances such as dusts (Table 2.1) may be inhaled. (Dusts may also be ingested as a second route of entry following inhaled particles returning via ciliary flow). Lead may be inhaled or absorbed through skin contamination. It may also be ingested secondary to, for example, nail-biting.

The effects on the body may be:

1. local irritant to the skin, eye or respiratory system;

2. allergy, usually of the skin or the respiratory tract;

3. systemic effect, toxicity of substance or metabolite.

The routes of inhalation, ingestion and absorption may not be related to the health effect. For example, the effect of the inhalation or skin absorption of solvents may manifest itself as neurological symptoms (drowsiness or dizziness) or liver disease.

Other factors influencing the effect of substances on workers include the individual worker's status in terms of age, sex, previous exposure, atopic state and general health.

STATISTICS RELATED TO OCCUPATIONAL DISEASES

These figures are available in the Health and Safety Executive Annual Report 1991–92 (HSC, 1992a) published by the Health and Safety Commission and can be used to identify some aspects of the relationship between work and health.

For example, we have mentioned mesothelioma. In 1982, 123 new claimants were awarded compensation under the Industrial Injuries and the Pneumoconiosis, Byssinosis and Miscellaneous Diseases Benefit Schemes. (Pneumoconiosis is a general term for lung diseases which includes coal workers' pneumoconiosis; byssinosis is a lung disease associated with textile working.)

In June 1991, 519 new claimants were awarded compensation under these schemes. This example illustrates the problem of work-related health effects that are not immediately obvious. Remember my earlier comment in this chapter about latency periods.

Occupational lung diseases

Statistics showing new claimants who have been awarded benefits for other occupational diseases show that in 1989:

Pneumoconiosis (except asbestosis)	437
Asbestosis	280
Byssinosis	15
Farmer's lung	13
Occupational asthma	220
Lung cancer (asbestos)	54
Lung cancer (other agents)	6
Bilateral pleural thickening	125

(HSE, 1991, p. 89)

Because of the latency effect, these claimants may no longer be working in the occupation during which they contracted the disease.

Occupational deafness

During the same year, 1989, 1506 claimants were awarded benefit for occupational deafness.

Table 2.1 Workplace hazards: Chemical

Workplace hazard	Example of type of job	Example of possible effect on health					
Chemical hazard		Poisoning	Dermatitis	Asthma	Lung disease	Cancer	Burns
Toxic substances	1 Chemical process worker	✓	✓	✓	✓	✓	✓
Solvents	2 Laboratory workers	✓	✓	✓	✓	✓	✓
Fibres	3 Food workers		✓	✓	✓		✓
Dusts	4 Fabric/clothes manufacturers			✓	✓		✓
	5 Electronic assembly workers	✓	✓	✓			✓
	6 Metal finishing workers	✓	✓	✓	✓		
	7 Lead workers	✓	✓	✓			
	8 Farm workers	✓	✓		✓	✓	
	9 Engineers			✓	✓		
	10 Welders	✓			✓		✓

Table 2.2 Workplace hazards: Physical

Workplace hazard	Example of type of job	Example of possible effect on health										
		Noise induced deafness	Vibration white finger	Blood diseases	Skin diseases	Cataracts	Impaired fertility	Other eye diseases	Hypoxia	Compression effects (joints CNS, ear)	Heat stroke	Hypothermia
Physical hazard												
e.g.												
1 Noise	1 Woodworkers (saws)	✓										
	2 Drinks manufacturers (bottling halls)	✓										
	3 Shipyard workers	✓										
	4 Metal workers	✓										
2 Vibration	5 Power tool workers		✓									
	6 Agricultural workers (chain saws)		✓									

Table 2.2 *continued*

Hazard	Workers					
3 Radiation (X and gamma radiation)	7a Health workers – technicians	✓	✓	✓		
	– dentists	✓	✓	✓		
	8 Nuclear energy workers	✓	✓	✓	✓	
	9 Industrial research & development workers	✓	✓	✓	✓	
– non-ionizing (ultra violet light, invisible light, infrared, radio frequency)	10 Laboratory workers	✓		✓		
	11 Beauty therapists	✓		✓		
	12 Welders (arc eye)			✓		
4 Abnormal pressure	13 Divers					✓
	14 Aviation workers					✓
5 Extremes of heat	15 Food workers (bakeries)					✓
6 Extremes of cold	16 Food workers (deep freezers)					✓

Table 2.3 Workplace hazards: Biological

Workplace hazard	Example of type of job	Example of possible effect on health		
		Infection	Allergy	Poisoning (Toxicity)
Biological hazard				
Micro-organisms	1 Health workers	✓	✓	✓
– bacteria	2 Laboratory workers	✓	✓	✓
– viruses	3 Teachers	✓		
– zoonoses (animal borne)	4 Child-care assistants	✓		
	5 Vets	✓	✓	✓
	6 Farm workers	✓	✓	
	7 Butchers	✓		
	8 Poultry workers		✓	Salmonella
	9 Sewage workers	✓		✓

Table 2.4 Workplace hazards: Ergonomic

Workplace hazard	Example of type of job	Back pain	WRULD*	Other musculo-skeletal disorder	Eye strain
Ergonomic hazard					
Manual handling	1 Health workers	✓			
Repetitive movements	2 Farmers	✓			
	3 Vets	✓			
Design of work station	4 Production-line workers	✓	✓	✓	
	5 Shelf fillers	✓		✓	
	6 Supermarket cashiers	✓	✓	✓	
	7 Food preparation	✓	✓	✓	✓
	- vegetable cleaning				
	- poultry workers				
Posture	8 Sedentary workers	✓		✓	
Visual display screens	9 VDU operators	✓	✓		✓

*Work Related Upper Limb Disorder

Table 2.5 Workplace hazards: Organizational

Workplace hazard	Example of type of job	Example of possible effect on health						
		Occupational stress	Digestive problems	Anxiety	Depression	Alcohol or drug abuse	Concentration problems	Personality change
Organization hazard	Could be any job where aspects of work organization or work station or task design can cause stress. These aspects include: 1 Working group dynamics 2 Shift patterns 3 Threat (real or not) of √ redundancy 4 Continuous change 5 Too much (or too little) responsibility 6 Fear or violence at work	√	√	√	√	√	√	√

Other occupational diseases

Other occupational diseases for which benefit may be payable include (HSC, 1991, p. 89):

	Numbers receiving disablement benefit 1989/90
Dermatitis	301
Tenosynovitis	423
Vibration White Finger	2601
Beat conditions	95
Viral hepatitis	1
Tuberculosis	0
Leptospirosis	2
Other infections	2
Poisonings	33
Occupational cancers	18
Other conditions	54
Total	3530

In order to obtain benefit, claimants must work, or have worked, in certain defined occupations and demonstrate a degree of disability related to the particular disease for which they are claiming. Claimants can find this a tedious process and, in some cases, trades-union support is enlisted.

It is not easy to be categorical about the direct effect of work on health; total benefit paid under these schemes does not reflect the real size of the problem. The references at the end of this chapter direct you to further reading in this area.

THE EFFECT OF WORK ON VULNERABLE GROUPS

Some occupational groups may be additionally challenged by the effect of work on health. These include pregnant women and people with disabilities. The effects of health on work are dealt with in the next chapter, but what about the relationship between work and pregnancy?

How may the work a woman does in pregnancy affect her health or that of the unborn child? Women are working longer into their pregnancies (Chamberlain, 1984). A survey carried out by Daniels (1980) and quoted by Chamberlain demonstrated that the percentage of women working in pregnancy had risen from 28% in 1946 to 48% in 1979 and that the percentage of those working after 30 weeks' gestation had risen from 10% in 1946 to 75% in 1979 (Chamberlain, 1984). This has implications from an occupational health perspective.

We have already discussed the general effects of work on health in terms of the effect of exposure to potentially hazardous substances. In the pregnant woman, this exposure may not only affect the individual but also her unborn child. The effects of physical hazards such as ionizing radiation have been known for some time (Bethell and Stewart [1975] in *Pregnant Women at Work* (ed.) G. Chamberlain) and point to the relationship between irradiation of the foetus and childhood leukaemia. The association is compounded by the fact that the foetus is at its most vulnerable in early pregnancy when the worker may be unaware that she is pregnant. Chemical hazards such as lead, mercury and solvents have been suspected of having reproductive effects for some time (Murray 1984 in *Pregnant Women at Work* (ed.) G. Chamberlain). Biological hazards may also affect the outcome of a pregnancy because of severe infections. Mamelle and Laumon (1984) in *Pregnant Women at Work* (ed.) G. Chamberlain have identified an association between occupational fatigue (which may be present in many jobs) and prematurity. They suggest that as many as 21% of premature births are caused by an occupational risk factor.

In compiling an occupational profile of a sample of pregnant women attending two booking clinics, Foster and Mitchell (1987) found that the women interviewed identified standing and lifting as the aspects of their work that gave them most concern. This sample was asked about their occupational exposure to agents such as dust, fume, noise, vibration, extremes of temperature, ionizing radiation, non-ionizing radiation and lifting and standing. The following table is reproduced from the 1987 report (Foster and Mitchell, 1987, p. 6). The table shows the reported exposure to potential workplace hazards as perceived by the pregnant women. The women were asked to rate exposures as low, medium or high. Perceived exposure to workplace hazards could have been in more than just one category: lifting and standing, for example, frequently occurred together. Perceptions of 'other' exposure related exclusively to stress.

Table 2.6 Repeated exposure to workplace hazards

	Low	Med	High	Total
Noise	19	8	0	27
Vibration	2	1	0	3
High temperature	6	2	1	9
Low temperature	4	0	1	5
Dust	4	0	0	4
Fume	4	1	0	5
Lifting	12	4	1	17
Standing	22	22	10	54
Ionizing radiation	1	0	0	1
Non-ironizing radiation	0	0	0	0
Other	10	1	0	11

The findings of the report were used to produce guidance for midwives and antenatal clinic staff (*Occupational   Health Aspects of Pregnancy* – leaflet MA6) in order that they may be more familiar with workplace factors which may influence the course of their client's pregnancy. This is an example of how non-occupational health specialists can become intermediaries in promoting occupational health and in widening the scope and effectiveness of their practice, ultimately benefiting their patients/clients.

CANCERS ASSOCIATED WITH OCCUPATION

Table 1 illustrating chemical hazards has suggested that some occupational exposure under certain conditions (circumstances of exposure, length of time exposed and concentration of substance) may lead to malignant disease. Some occupational cancers have been recognized for many years: Harrington and Gill (1992) point out that Rehn identified the risk of bladder tumours in dye workers at the end of the nineteenth century. Other cancers occurring among occupational groups include skin cancers in farmers or seamen, lung cancers associated with some chromium compounds, liver cancer in vinyl-chloride production workers, nasal sinus cancer in woodworkers, and bone-marrow cancer associated with health-care workers.

The aetiology of the disease is not always well defined and this, coupled with the latency period, means that an immediate association may not be apparent. Harrington and Gill (1992) list the characteristics of occupational carcinogens as:

1. They tend to occur earlier than 'spontaneous' tumours of the same size.

2. Exposure to the putative agent is repeated but not necessarily continuous.

3. The latent period is 10–40 years.

4. The tumours are often multiple in a given organ.

5. Despite widely differing estimates of the proportion of all cancers caused by occupation, the true figure probably lies in the range of 3%–8%.

(Harrington and Gill, 1992, p. 228)

Harrington and Gill also point out the problem of multiple chemical exposure and the effect of synergy in the relationship between exposure to asbestos and smoking.

HOW CAN THIS CHAPTER IMPROVE PRACTICE IN DELIVERING HEALTH CARE?

This chapter has attempted to give a broad picture of the effects of work on health. Whichever your area of practice, the relationship between work and health should be considered when drawing up a care programme for your patient/client.

I hope to have encouraged you to add this dimension when assessing, planning, implementing and evaluating your patients'/clients' care programmes. In the practice of clinical nursing, the effect of work on health may not only contribute to disease but may also affect rehabilitation and recovery. In preventive and promotional work, a knowledge of the workplace will be useful when providing clients with information from which they may make choices. When planning research studies it will be useful to know if 'occupation' could be a variable to be considered. For those of you who undergo midwifery or health-visitor training, I hope this chapter will have given you some insight into the problems of combining work with pregnancy. Some of you may develop an interest in occupational health and I hope that this chapter may have provided a starting point.

FURTHER READING

Notes on the Diagnosis of Occupational Diseases (prescribed under industrial injuries Provisions of Social Security Act 1975). Department of Social Security, HMSO, London, UK.

Barlow, S.M. and Sullivan, F.M. (1982) *Reproductive Hazards of Industrial Chemicals*, Academic Press, London.

Hunter, D. (1969) *The Diseases of Occupations* (4th edn), English Universities Press Ltd, UK.

Slaney, B. (ed.) (1980) *Occupational Health Nursing*, Croom Helm, London.

Waldron, H.A. (1989) *Occupational Health Practice*, Butterworth, UK.

Waldron, H.A. (1990) *Lecture Notes on Occupational Health*, Blackwell Scientific Publications, Oxford.

REFERENCES

Bamford, M. (1992) personal communication.

Bethell, J.F. and Stewart, A.M. (1975) The hazards of work in pregnancy, in Chamberlain, G. (ed.) *Pregnant Women at Work*, The Royal Society of Medicine and Macmillan, London, p. 28.

Chamberlain, G. (ed.) (1984) *Pregnant Women at Work*, The Royal Society of Medicine and Macmillan, London.

Foster, A. and Mitchell, M.A.R. (1987) *An Occupational Profile on 292 Women Presenting at Two Antenatal Booking Clinics in North London*, Health and Safety Executive Research Report, HSE, London.

Harrington, J.M. and Gill, F.S. (1992) *Occupational Health*, (3rd edn), Blackwell Scientific, London.

Health and Safety Commission (1992) *Annual Report 1991/92*, HMSO, London.

Health and Safety Executive (1989) *Occupational Health Aspects of Pregnancy*, M50, 1/89, (MA6), HMSO, London.

Health and Safety Executive (1992a) *Your Patients and Their Work*, Employment Department Group publications, UK C600, 11/92, HMSO, London.

Health and Safety Executive (1992b) *Manual Handling – Guidance on Regulations*, HMSO, London.

Health and Safety Executive (1992c) *Occupational Health Provision at Work*, Research Report by IFF Research, unpublished HSE report.

HMSO (1975) *Social Security Act 1975*, HMSO, London.

Mamelle, N. and Laumon, B. (1984) Occupational fatigue and preterm birth, in Chamberlain, G. (ed.) *Pregnant Women at Work*, The Royal Society of Medicine and the Macmillan, London, pp. 105–15.

Murray, R. (1984) The hazards of work in pregnancy, in Chamberlain, G. (ed.) *Pregnant Women at Work*, The Royal Society of Medicine and the Macmillan Press Ltd., London, p. 31.

Schilling, R.S.F. (1981) *Occupational Health Practice* (2nd edn), Butterworth, London.

3

The effects of health on work

Cynthia Atwell

INTRODUCTION

The effects of 'health on work' and 'work on health' are synonymous with each other. In considering a person's suitability for
employment, the health status must be assessed and matched to
the requirements of the job, taking account of the physical and
psychological demands of the work. There are many situations
where individuals are unnecessarily refused employment on
health grounds because the assessment has been made on health
status alone, with no reference to the demands of the job to be
carried out.

It has been estimated that over one million people are absent
from work each day because of sickness or other cause (ACAS,
1985), at enormous cost to business and society. Furthermore, the
pressure put on to employment pension schemes for 'ill-health'
retirements can be quite considerable, more so in times of economic recession when employers consider that any attempt at
redeployment or rehabilitation in the workplace is too costly. The
Employment Protection Act (1978) and the Disabled Persons
(Employment) Act 1944 and 1958 are statutes introduced to protect employees from unfair dismissal and discrimination arising
from ill health or disability. The Health of the Nation (1992)
discusses the major causes of death in our nation and sets targets
for reducing this in specific areas.

It is important that these issues are considered in relation to
an individual's ability to do a particular job. Little attention is
paid to the importance of health and work, when it is a fact that
half our nation is at work, providing the economic and social

support needed for those unable to support themselves and their families because of ill health or disability.

FITNESS/SUITABILITY FOR WORK

Pre-employment health/medical assessment is carried out by most large and medium-sized employers. It is either provided by an in-house occupational health service, a local GP or through other private health schemes. Potential employees may be required to complete a pre-employment questionnaire which asks a series of questions about health status, requiring a yes/no answer; undergo a health screening by an occupational health nurse or a medical examination by the company doctor. Health assessment procedures should be suitable for the organization and the individual's needs to meet specific criteria and not purely as a 'routine', without real purpose.

Times when health assessment is necessary will vary but as a general rule this will be: pre-employment; periodic for those who work with known hazards and to comply with legal requirements; following illness or injury; monitoring those with known health problems to ensure their condition does not worsen; prior to job change or promotion and as part of a health-promotion programme.

Why then is health assessment necessary? The answer must be addressed before such assessments are carried out:

- Information obtained will form a baseline of the standard of health for the individual, which will act as a measure for future assessment. Baseline information and records will form vital epidemiological data, which should be used to look at the health status of groups of workers to develop health policies and standards for the workforce;
- To screen out those who may be unsuitable for a particular job;
- To ensure that those who have known health problems are not exposed to hazardous work situations likely to exacerbate the condition, for example someone with asthma being placed in a job working with known asthma-causing agents;
- To assess a person's working capacity and to match this to a suitable job;

- To enable the employee to enter the company pension/superannuation scheme and/or for insurance purposes;
- To protect the product, as in the case of food production where the worker must be free from infections which are transmissible through food;
- As part of the organization's overall policy for positive health promotion.

PRE-EMPLOYMENT SCREENING PROCEDURES

Pre-employment health screening by nurses and doctors should only be done for specific reasons (Braddick, Atwell and Tar-Ching, 1992). Screening procedures for pre-employment health assessment need to be standardized and parameters set for acceptance or rejection, depending on the type of work. This type of assessment is quite within the capabilities of a suitably qualified nurse, provided the nurse is educated and trained to carry out specific procedures, is competent to do so and has detailed knowledge and understanding of the job and the hazards involved. Qualified occupational health nurses (OHNs) come into this category and in most organizations health assessments form a major role for the OHN.

Before embarking on a screening procedure it will be necessary to know what the job is and to have a job specification. The screening required will be dictated by the needs of the job and individual and may contain some or all of the following:

General observations of the person

Mobility, posture, evidence of disability, height/body mass; general appearance and standard of hygiene, condition of skin; evidence of breathing difficulties.

Height/weight ratio

Some companies set standards for height/weight. This will be particularly important where someone is working in a confined space or where high levels of activity are required in the job. Height can often be a factor to consider for ambulance/fire personnel, where they are required to work in fairly restricted vehicles, or rescue situations which could lead to back pain and cervical-spine problems.

Weight standards cannot be set in isolation, nor should they be too rigid. Body mass generally will be the deciding factor and must be compared with the height and general health status of the individual.

Vision screening

Visual acuity, both distance and near vision, will need to be assessed, particularly where good vision is required for safe working. Visual fields should also be checked where good peripheral vision is necessary, for example working with robot machinery, moving vehicles, chemicals and molten substances. Employees who have tunnel vision and are working in such areas may put other employees at risk. Also included would be drivers of Large Goods Vehicles (LGV), Public Service Vehicles (PSV), cranes and fork lift trucks.

Testing visual distance of 26 inches is carried out for persons employed on Visual Display Units (VDUs) not because VDUs cause problems but because those working on VDUs for the first time may experience difficulties from a previously undiagnosed visual problem which VDU work may highlight. The Health and Safety (Display Screen Equipment) Regulations 1992 (HSE, 1992) require employers to offer vision screening, or eyesight tests by a qualified optician to all those who are regular VDU users, at pre-employment stage and at regular intervals thereafter. Testing for depth perception will be required for some types of work such as driving and where it is necessary for the individual to judge distance and space relationships.

Colour perception may be important for safety reasons such as hazard warnings, cable and wiring and pipelines. Some work may involve colour matching and dyeing where colour differentiation is important. Areas of medical diagnosis and chemical analysis may present difficulties and transport-signalling systems may use colour codes. In assessing colour vision it is important to select the right test for the particular situation. Special tests can be set which are based on the occupation, requiring the potential employee to carry out a job test. In the past, judgements have been wrongly made on requirements for colour vision. People have been rejected for 'colour blindness' based on too harsh standards, where other methods of identification could be used, for example for drivers, where the traffic-signal sequence is used rather than relying solely on the colour of the lights. Edwards *et al.* (1988) states that 8% of men and 0.2% of women have defective colour vision, a statistic that must be considered to avoid unnecessary discrimination.

Examination of the ear

Examination of the ear with an auroscope will be necessary for those people who are to be employed in work that requires a level of hygiene to protect the product, such as food handlers, or medical products such as sterile dressings.

The examiner will need to ensure that the ear is free from obvious infection and that the eardrum is intact with no evidence of discharge. If the eardrum is obliterated by a build-up of wax, this will need to be removed. This may require the person to be referred to their own GP for this to be done and therefore the examination will not be complete; the individual will need to be seen again at a later date.

Hearing loss may be associated with disease of the middle ear or be present since birth. Tinnitus (ringing in the ears) is often associated with hearing loss. Unless hearing is a prime requirement for the job, such as in work requiring detailed communication skills or for safety reasons, people with hearing difficulty should not be barred from employment. There are many aids available to help people with hearing difficulties, such as hearing loops, telephones with amplified handsets, inductive couplers linked to specially adapted hearing aids, visual hazard-warning systems: all these should be considered to assist employment.

A history of balance disorders (vertigo) may be caused by a number of different conditions and can bar people from certain occupations such as working at heights, vocational driving and diving or flying where there are changes in barometric pressure. However, each case must be assessed taking account of all the factors when deciding on suitability. Examination of the ear requires special skills and it will be important for the nurse to ensure that he/she is suitably trained and experienced. The auroscope and audiometer will be the main pieces of equipment used.

Audiometry may be carried out on individuals who are to be employed in potentially noisy areas. The results will form a baseline against which further tests can be compared, especially where a hearing-conservation programme is being introduced to comply with the Noise at Work Regulations (HSE, 1989).

Blood-pressure estimation

This should be recorded routinely at pre-employment health assessment, as abnormalities are easily recognized and can be treated. Hypertension (raised blood pressure) may be a sign of early cardiovascular or kidney disease and needs further investigation. It is important to remember that anxiety can cause a slight rise in blood pressure and must be taken into account at the pre-employment stage when the person may well be anxious. Well-controlled hypertensive people can be employed in many occupations, particularly if they are controlled on diet only or with mild doses of diuretic preparations. Those controlled with stronger drugs may have problems with side-effects and this will need to be taken into account. Vocational driving is one of the occupations where strict standards are set. Raffle's *Medical Aspects of Fitness to Drive* (1985) advises that a person with a casual blood pressure of 200/110 or over should not hold a vocational driving licence.

Urine-testing

As with blood pressure, this should also be a routine part of the assessment. It will pick up early diagnosis of diabetes mellitus and kidney disease, both of which may have practical implications for employment.

Some organizations have introduced substance-abuse policies which require employees to be tested for drug and/or alcohol abuse. This can be carried out by urine-testing and necessitates special sampling, conveying and testing systems. The main purpose for substance-abuse testing is to safeguard other employees, the company and its assets, the general public and the environment. This may form part of pre-employment screening as well as being on-going.

Lung function testing

This will be required for those who will be working in potentially dusty environments, with asthma-causing agents such as isocyanates, flour or grain dust, in confined spaces where there may be a requirement to wear breathing apparatus, for example for sewer workers or mines rescuers, and in work where a high level of activity is a requirement of the job, particularly if the potential employee has a history of respiratory disease and/or is a heavy smoker with evidence of reduced lung capacity.

Various tests may be undertaken. The most commonly used are the estimation of forced vital capacity (FVC) and forced expiratory volume in one second (FEV1) which can be measured using a portable spirometer. This will also print out the data which can be kept on record for future comparison. There is also a peak flow meter (PFM) which is used over a period of time to detect evidence of abnormal function. The individual is required to blow into the PFM at regular intervals over a period of time; then the results are traced in the form of a graph to see if there are specific times of the day/night/week when there is a significant reduction in lung function. All these tests require specialist knowledge and training to ensure they are carried out and interpreted correctly.

Chest radiography may also be required but this will be the remit of the medical adviser and will normally be arranged through a local hospital or clinic.

Electrocardiography (ECG)

This should only be necessary when a full medical assessment is required and should be under the auspices of the medical adviser. Where the nurse is required to carry out this procedure, they must ensure they are competent to do so.

Blood tests

There are a few occasions when blood-testing is required during pre-employment screening, although it is widely used as a means of assessing exposure to certain hazardous agents, such as lead, during employment. Blood-testing to assess hepatitis 'B' antibody status for health-care workers is widely carried out in order to establish the need for hepatitis 'B' vaccination. In some cases, antigen status is also measured, particularly on those health-care workers such as surgeons and midwives who, if carriers of the virus, may infect those in their care.

The whole of screening for hepatitis 'B' is controversial and remains under discussion within the professions. Therefore on this matter the nurse must be mindful of the ethical dilemma and ensure that if they are expected to undertake such screening, they are fully aware of the procedure and implications and the need for strict confidentiality.

SPECIFIC HEALTH ISSUES AND EFFECTS ON EMPLOYMENT

When assessing someone's suitability to do a job there must be assessment of the person's functional ability to do it, taking note of the individual's capacity and matching that to its demands. There will be a need for the person carrying out the assessment to have detailed knowledge of the work and tasks involved, the general working environment and the potential health effects of any hazardous substances being used and the methods for controlling those hazards. There are many conditions that, in the past, have been stigmatized, so much so that people with these health problems have been discriminated against. In the following section some of these problems will be discussed.

Epilepsy

There is still no definitive epidemiological evidence available to show the causes of epilepsy. Many people will relate it to a particular illness, injury or event in their lives which 'brought it on'. Historically, people with epilepsy have been disadvantaged and if they declared their condition at pre-employment health assessment, they would not be employed. Epilepsy which developed during employment usually meant the individual could be dismissed on health grounds or forced to take early retirement.

If epilepsy is declared at pre-employment health assessment then it will be important to establish the details of the job and any potential hazards. Contact should be made with the employee's GP or consultant in order to ascertain details of the person's condition. It will be necessary to obtain written consent to do this, as laid down under the Access to Medical Reports Act 1988 (DofE, 1987). No attempt should be made to advise on suitability for employment without a full health history from the person's own GP.

The Road Traffic Act (1972 and 1974) does not allow a person to hold a Large Goods Vehicle (LGV) licence if they have had an epileptic attack since attaining the age of five. This also applies to Public Service Vehicle drivers (PSV), all other vocational drivers, train drivers, airline pilots, crane operators and fork-lift-truck drivers.

The safety of the individual and others will need to be considered. Other types of unsuitable work are jobs involving climbing and/or working at heights such as steeple-jacks, scaffolders, firemen/women; work in isolation, particularly if it is maintenance or electrical work which requires the person to work with high-voltage electricity and/or unguarded machinery.

The majority of people with epilepsy are capable of undertaking most types of employment. There are, however, a minority who may have additional disabilities which may be physical or associated with learning difficulties and require a more sheltered work environment with close supervision and major restrictions. This should only be the case when all details of the individual's medical history have been examined and an informed judgement made on the need for this course of action.

Many people do not disclose the fact that they have a history of seizures or convulsions when they apply for a job or during pre-employment health assessment. This could cause major problems for the employer and the employee as it could be contravening Section 7 of the Health and Safety at Work Act (HMSO, 1974) which requires the employee to ensure the health and safety of him/herself and of others. Also, non-disclosure may negate any insurance cover that has been provided. The attitude of the employer will be a factor that affects disclosure. If the employer has a well-publicised, positive employment policy, which does not unnecessarily discriminate against people with epilepsy, then the potential employee is likely to have the confidence to declare the disability. The responsibility for the employment of a person with epilepsy is that of the employer. The decision must be based on sound medical advice, together with sound knowledge of the work and workplace hazards; anything less is unfair to both employee and employer.

Diabetes mellitus

Diabetes can be classified into two main categories:

1. Insulin-dependent diabetes, which is caused by damage to the islets of Langerhans, resulting in insufficient production of insulin to support metabolism. It can occur at any age but is most commonly diagnosed before the age of 20.
2. Non-insulin-dependent diabetes usually occurs after the age of 30. Its cause in most cases is unknown and the majority of diabetics come into this category.

Diabetes remains poorly understood and those with the condition experience difficulty in gaining employment mainly because of the fears of employers. Provided the potential employee is properly assessed and the hazards of the proposed work known and understood, these fears are largely unjustified. A small proportion of people with diabetes develop long-term complications, usually after many years. These are visual complications such as cataract and retinopathy, which can lead to blindness; and leg and foot ulceration which may, in severe cases, lead to amputation of the affected limb. There is also increased evidence that diabetics are at higher risk of cardiovascular disease such as heart attacks and strokes.

When assessing a person with insulin-dependent diabetes, a full, detailed history will be required and therefore contact will need to be made with the person's GP and/or consultant in order to obtain the full picture. Suitability must be based on the requirements of the job in relation to how well-controlled the individual is and the ability of the person to understand their health status and the likely complications.

Irregular work patterns as with shiftwork has in the past given cause for concern when employing a person with diabetes. For the individual who is well-controlled, who can carry out their own regular blood-glucose estimate and understand how to maintain and adjust their insulin treatment, shiftwork should not be an insurmountable problem. One development that may pose a problem is the introduction of shorter shift cycles: for example, cycles that change every 48 hours, which would not give sufficient time for insulin adjustment.

The major concern of everyone in employing someone with diabetes is that the person may have hypoglycaemic attacks which can cause the person to be confused and/or lose consciousness. Most insulin-dependent diabetics have ample warnings of impending hypoglycaemia and can take preventive steps in the form of glucose, therefore avoiding the situation. The risk of hypoglycaemia has often been exaggerated but must be a factor when considering suitability for employment. It is advisable to ensure that a person with diabetes does not work alone for long periods; it will be necessary to consider the dangers involved when working at heights and with potentially dangerous machinery. The guiding rule must be to assess whether or not the outcome of a hypoglycaemic attack will endanger the life of the individual or others.

As with epilepsy, insulin-dependent diabetics are not permitted to hold a vocational driver's licence (LGV and PSV). The situation for existing drivers who subsequently develop diabetes will depend on the type of diabetes, how well-controlled the individual is and whether the licence was issued before 1 January 1983. A vocational driver who is well-controlled with diet and/or oral drugs, and without complications, will normally be permitted to keep their licence.

Other occupations which are barred are the police, the fire service, being an airline pilot and train driving, although the latter has been relaxed to allow well-controlled, non-insulin-dependent diabetics to drive trains, provided they are closely monitored and remain controlled.

Once the person with diabetes has been employed it will be necessary for them to be given support and facilities in order for them to be able to carry out blood-glucose testing and administer their treatment at the place of work. Arrangements will also need to be made to ensure that adequate facilities are available for regular meal breaks. Dietary requirements will need to be discussed with the catering manager where meals are provided and available at the workplace.

It is essential that every individual person is assessed on their own merits. This requires a full investigation into the health history of the individual through liaison with the GP and/or consultant. Only when this has been done and matched to the requirements of the proposed occupation can a proper informed decision be made on the individual's suitability.

Cardiovascular impairment

This may be as a result of congenital disease or acquired, as with myocardial infarction, hypertension and ischaemic heart disease (IHD). The latter is preventable through the cessation of smoking, increased activity through exercise and the provision of a healthy diet. Major innovations in treatment, including surgical intervention, has improved the quality and quantity of life for many of those who would previously either have not been able to work or would have been forced to retire from active employment because of their poor level of health.

Ischaemic heart disease is responsible for approximately 25% of male deaths between the ages of 40 and 59 years and is much greater in social classes 4 and 5 (Shaper *et al.*, 1984). Over the past few years much attention has been paid to the prevention of IHD and many employers have embarked on health-education programmes in an attempt to improve the health and productivity of their employees. The development of non-smoking policies, encouraging exercise by the provision of facilities at work and improved diet from canteen facilities have all made a contribution.

Assessment of the potential employee who has had cardiovascular impairment will need to be thorough and in liaison with the person's GP and/or consultant. The history of the disease and its onset will be vital, together with an informed prognosis. Many employers remain concerned about employing people with 'heart trouble' because of the unpredictable and often devastating consequences of someone collapsing at work and the employer's concern about their legal liability. For this reason there are often artificial restrictions placed on people which helps neither the employer or employee. Work restrictions are placed on airline pilots, LGV and PSV drivers, train drivers, police and fire officers. They are rarely allowed to return to work following a myocardial infarction, as in most cases the risk of sudden collapse at work would be disastrous. Work with solvents such as trichlorethylene or carbon tetrachloride may cause sudden irregular heart-beat and for this reason may be restricted. Proper workplace control of these substances is a requirement under the Control of Substances Hazardous to Health Regulations 1988 (COSHH) (HMSO, 1987) and therefore should be less of a restriction if these regulations have been implemented.

Most problems arise in employing people with IHD, particularly those who have been employed and wish to return to their former occupation. It will be necessary to ensure a full assessment is made of the employee, including exercise-tolerance testing. If there are no undue symptoms, then return to work should be arranged in consultation with the employee and the employee's GP and manager. The return may need to be phased either on reduced hours initially and/or changed duties, until such time as the employee feels able to carry out the full range of duties. The return-to-work rehabilitation programme and placement should always be developed to meet the needs of the individual and the employing organization; every programme will be different. One of the main problems for someone returning to work after a cardiac event is anxiety caused by the fear of a reoccurrence. This situation needs careful handling and understanding and the employee will need support and counselling at work. The anxiety may be partly a result of family concerns or pressure from work colleagues. All those concerned about the welfare of the employee will need reassurance in order to help them give the needed support.

GASTRO-INTESTINAL DYSFUNCTION

Diseases of the digestive tract are responsible for a considerable number of lost working days. Conditions that are common causes of absence are gastric ulcers, gastroenteritis and irritable bowel syndrome. Few gastrointestinal conditions would be a bar to employment, apart from those who may have undergone major surgery, thus reducing the individual's working capacity. Those who have had major surgery may have difficulties with work which involves heavy lifting, and some shift work. Each person must be fully assessed. The assessment should be made after consultation with the individual's GP and/or consultant in order to gain a full history of the condition and details of any surgical interventions that may have been carried out.

The employee may require advice on diet and rest-breaks at work. This will be necessary where they will be working varied shift patterns in order to ensure that they receive regular meals. Employees who have temporary or permanent stomas (ileostomy, colostomy) should be able to carry out most forms of employment depending on the reason for the surgery and their subsequent general state of health. Facilities for changing appliances and dressings will be required. These should be private and include facilities for washing. Where an occupational-health department is available, it may be appropriate for these facilities to be available there. This would also give the individual access to professional advice and help when required.

Employees who complain of irritable bowel syndrome (IBS) may have frequent short spells of absence from work. Their symptoms include diarrhoea and abdominal pains which can be distressing for the sufferer and cause concern to work colleagues. The condition is often predisposed to an anxiety state or major stressful incident, which is sometimes caused by the work. People with IBS need to be referred to their GP for investigation and treatment and to avoid excessive stressful situations.

Skin care

The skin is the largest organ of the body. It acts as a barrier against infection and is a tough, resilient cushion that protects internal tissues. It helps to regulate body temperature and it is also a sense organ which responds to pain, heat, cold, touch and pressure. Because the skin acts as a protective barrier, it is greatly abused and neglected and susceptible to disease and injury. We challenge our skin in everyday life by exposing it to excessive sunlight (when we have the opportunity!) and by placing our hands in all types of cleaning agents and chemicals, without considering the long-term effects of these actions on its health. It is not until something goes wrong that we consider 'skin care'.

It is important for the employee to understand the relevance of good skin care. Correct hand-washing ensures the skin has been properly cleaned. Drying the skin with suitable disposable towels or hot air dryers and then the application of a moisturing 'after work' cream to replace the natural oils that will have been lost through all these activities ensures good care.

Many occupations involving the handling of degreasing and sensitizing agents will present problems to someone with a skin condition. When assessing the suitability of someone for employment with these agents it will be necessary to pay special attention to the health of the employee's skin. Those with a history of skin disease such as eczema, psoriasis and dermatitis will need to be carefully assessed and a detailed history obtained from their GP. Once this is done, an informed decision can be made, bearing in mind the hazards of the particular job. With the introduction of recent health and safety legislation, control measures should be such that most people will not be at risk, but those with a history of sensitization may be unsuitable for employment with known sensitizing agents such as epoxy resins and nickel. The key to healthy skin is to educate the employee about skin care and ensure that where necessary, suitable protective clothing is provided and worn correctly.

Mental health

Psychiatric illness remains a taboo subject in society, largely because of ignorance and fear. Health professionals should be aware of this and help to educate people in order to alleviate these prejudices. Mental illness can effect people of all ages, occupations and social groups. It is often a barrier to progression and viewed as a basic weakness of the individual to cope with 'life'. Only a small proportion of people who become mentally ill will suffer long-term effects likely to make them difficult to employ. Most people will make a full recovery with no reoccurrence. In some cases, gaining employment (or retaining the previous job) acts as part of the healing and rehabilitation process and should be encouraged.

There are many different types of mental illness and it is not intended to discuss them in detail in this chapter. However, alcohol and substance dependency are two problems that require further discussion, as these present the employer with great difficulties for the health and safety of both the dependent employee and other employees.

It has been estimated that in the UK between 8 to 14 million working days each year are lost because of alcohol misuse, at a cost to industry of £1.6 million pounds (WHO, 1992). It has been estimated that 1 in 10 employees in Britain have drink-related problems (IRS, 1992) and that a significant number of people who abuse drugs are in employment.

The taking of drugs, either therapeutic or addictive, brings about major changes in behaviour which affects an individual's ability to carry out a job safely and efficiently. People taking tranquillizers pose a major problem as they are more numerous; sedatives and hypnotics are also widely used. Most of these drugs reduce attention and cause short-term memory loss. Contrary to popular belief, people who use illegal drugs such as heroin or cocaine can still be in full-time employment. The employment of people with chronic alcohol or drug use/abuse problems is not recommended. Individuals should be advised to seek help at an early stage of their illness. However, those who have a history of drug/alcohol abuse should not be automatically rejected; many are successfully treated and do not relapse.

Because of concern about the effects of both alcohol and drugs in the workplace, many large organizations have introduced pre-employment drug/alcohol screening to preclude the employment of regular users. This screening has been introduced in major organizations involved with the production, handling and transportation of highly toxic substances, in order to protect the health and safety of the individual, co-workers and of course the general public and environment, who would be at risk if a major disaster occurred. Many other organizations are considering this action, particularly those involved with transport. The ethics of this type of screening must be considered and it should only be carried out with the full knowledge of the individual. Special arrangements will need to be set up in order to safeguard the authenticity of the samples and the reliability of the test results. Confidentiality of the results must also be assured.

Some companies have introduced substance-abuse policies as a means of encouraging early recognition and treatment of those with alcohol/drug-related problems in employment. This is to be applauded and encouraged, as it is a means of controlling any problems before they get out of hand.

Alcohol/drug dependency will not be readily identified on pre-employment health assessment. Most people would not declare this problem on a questionnaire and would not necessarily confide in the doctor or nurse at examination, so it would be appropriate to contact the individual's GP, provided consent is given, if there is cause for concern.

All potential employees with a history of mental illness should be assessed in the same way as for any other condition. People should not be rejected solely on the grounds of mental illness: they must be considered on their merits, experience and abilities. Limitations should be recognized and matched to the requirements of the proposed job. (See Chapter Five for additional reading on aspects of mental health and work.)

Infectious conditions

Infections in the workplace have always been a cause for concern, particularly the common cold and influenza which can rapidly devastate a working population and therefore affect productivity. Rubella is also feared among those employers with high numbers of women employees and the risk of infection being contracted at work by those women who are in the first trimester of pregnancy. This can be a significant problem for those women employed in teaching, health care, child minding, etc., where they may have contact with children who have rubella. These women should be screened for rubella antibodies and those who are negative should be offered vaccination.

Blood borne infections – human immunodeficiency virus (HIV) and hepatitis 'B'

The most significant infectious disease today is that of (HIV). It causes a great deal of concern for the employer, employees and the HIV-positive employee in the workplace. Most of these concerns are without foundation and caused through ignorance and prejudice about how the virus is transmitted. Many people still believe that the virus is transmitted through casual contact and the prejudice is enhanced by the fact that the virus is most prevalent among certain groups of people, therefore fuelling these prejudices. The latest figures showing the incidence of HIV infection indicate that there is an increase in HIV positivity among the heterosexual community, proving that it is not the 'group' that is the risk, but the 'behaviour' of people. No other health problem has caused such fear and anxiety in modern times.

In the vast majority of jobs there is no risk of HIV infection. Even in work where the virus or material which could contain the virus is handled, there appears to be little risk to those who have been exposed; and taking account of the need for safe working practices the virus can be handled relatively safely (McEvoy *et al.*, 1987).

The most important factor about HIV is one of confidentiality. Information gained through pre-employment health assessment must not be disclosed to the employer without the employee's consent. The nurse is in an ideal situation to help and support the HIV-positive employee through counselling and education. If the employee subsequently develops acquired immune deficiency syndrome (AIDS) the nurse must ensure that the employee receives the same support, treatment and care as any other employee with a life-threatening disease. Redeployment to less demanding work may have to be considered as the disease progresses. Every effort must be made to keep the employee in active employment for as long as they wish and the condition allows.

There continues to be much debate about whether health-care workers such as surgeons and midwives should be routinely screened for HIV, in order to protect their patients who may be at risk during surgical procedures or delivery, from accidental exposure. At present, all health-care workers who undertake surgical procedures which are high risk are expected to take special measures to ensure they do not transmit the virus to their patients. This usually means redeployment to another field of medicine for the unfortunate surgeon.

Hepatitis 'B' (HBV) is a more significant occupational risk for those working in health care. The majority of health-care workers need to be protected with Hepatitis 'B' vaccination which should be offered at pre-employment stage. The risk of the employee transmitting the virus to patients and clients is the same as for HIV, although the HBV is far more infectious and those health-care workers involved with surgical procedures should be redeployed away from direct blood contact with the patient.

Each month there is new information about HIV and HBV and it is important that health-care workers keep up-to-date with these developments. Good communications should be established with the regional virology laboratory and the consultant in public health medicine to ensure the latest information and advice is available.

Women's health

Women are frequently discriminated against in employment. Assumptions are made about their ability to work alongside male colleagues, without any substantial evidence.

There are certain times in a woman's life when there may be some difficulties, such as during pregnancy, menopause and, for some, before and during menstruation, a symptom known

as premenstrual syndrome (PMS). None of this should be a
to employment.

For the pregnant woman, a few specific hazards exist such as
working with chemicals like lead and mercury (this is discussed
in more detail in Chapter Two). A woman should not be rejected
for employment just because she is pregnant; alternative employment should be considered.

PMS includes symptoms of headaches, depression, anxiety
and severe breast soreness. During menstruation, some women
experience painful abdominal cramps which can be very debilita-
ting. The majority of women undergo the menopause without
any problems; some experience symptoms of 'hot flushes', sweats
and memory-retention difficulties. In severe cases, all these
symptoms may cause absenteeism from work. The nurse's role
is to recognize these problems and assist with counselling.
Women with severe problems should be encouraged to seek
help and treatment from their GP, as all these symptoms are
controllable. Advice on diet, exercise and sleep should also be
given and, when necessary, rest periods arranged for the
employee.

Disability and employment

Many people with disabilities do not need any special assistance
in order to gain employment. All they need is the opportunity to
be able to prove their capabilities. The employer with a positive
attitude towards employing disabled people will find that they
are able to perform as well as an 'able-bodied' person, given the
same opportunities. Assessment of any person for employment
must be based on a philosophy of 'ability' rather than concentrat-
ing on the 'disability'.

Disabled people are frequently discriminated against because
employers and their medical advisers are too cautious and place
unnecessary restrictions on their work; this makes it impossible
for the disabled person to be integrated into the workforce. If a
disabled person has the required qualifications, experience and
ability and there is no risk to health and safety, either to themselves or other fellow workers, they should be treated in the
same way as any other applicant.

In order to comply with the requirements of the Disabled
Persons (Employment) Acts 1944 and 1958 in helping people into

employment, the Acts provide that employers of more than 20 people should employ a quota of registered disabled people. At present this quota is set at 3% of the workforce.

In 1992 new developments took place for Employment Disability Services with the introduction of specialist local teams called Placing, Assessment and Counselling Teams (PACTs). PACTs have taken over the functions previously carried out by Disablement Resettlement Officers, the Disablement Advisory Service and the Employment Rehabilitation Service. The people who are available to advise employers and people with disabilities are now called Disability Employment Advisers (DEAs) and can be contacted through local job centres. PACTs will be available to give advice on recruitment and training and on retention of those who become disabled while in employment. They will also give advice and information about the special services available and advise on the quota scheme.

There are some occasions when a disabled person may require adaptations to be made to the workplace or require special aids to help them. Practical help on this, including grants and equipment, is available through PACTs.

Nurses must be mindful of the needs of disabled people and ensure they give the necessary advice and support to allow their integration into the workplace. A prime function will be one of educating the employer about the positive advantages of employing people with disabilities, both to the individual and the employing organization. Regular contact should be maintained with PACTs through the Occupational Health Service and personnel departments.

An information pack about the function of PACTs is available by contacting:
Employment Service Disability Services Branch
DS1, Level 3
Steel City House, c/o Rockingham House
123 West Street
Sheffield S1 4ER

USEFUL ADDRESSES

British Epilepsy Association
Anstey House,
40 Hanover Square

Leeds LS3 1BE (0532) 439393

also

92–94 Tooley Street,
London SE1 9SH 071–403 4111

British Diabetic Association
1 Queen Ann Street
London W1M 0DD 071–323 1531

The National Association for Mental Health (MIND)
22 Harley Street,
London W1N 2ED 071–637 0741

also

23 St Mary Street,
Cardiff CF1 2AA (0222) 395123

National Schizophrenia Fellowship
28 Castle Street,
Kingston upon Thames
Surrey KT1 1SS 081–547 3937

London School of Hygiene and Tropical Medicine
Department of Public Health and Policy
Keppel Street,
London WC1E 7HT 071–636 8636

Department of Health AIDS Unit,
Friars House
157–168 Blackfriars Road
London SE1 8EU 071–972 2000

Terrence Higgins Trust
BM/AIDS
London WC1N 3XX
Helpline 071–242 1010

National AIDS Trust
Room 1403 Euston Tower
286 Euston Road

London NW1 3DN
071–388 1188 ext. 3200

Local Health Authority,
Department of Public Health and/or Communicable Diseases
(see local telephone directory)

REFERENCES

Advisory Conciliation and Advisory Service (ACAS) (1985) Advisory booklet number 5, *Absence.*

Braddick, M.R., Atwell, C.P. and Aw Tar-Ching (1992) Audit of pre-employment health assessment in the National Health Service. *Journal of the Society of Occupational Medicine,* **42**, 36–8.

Department of Employment (1987) *Access to Medical Reports Act 1988,* HMSO, London.

Department of Employment, *Disabled Persons (Employment) Act 1944 and 1958,* HMSO, London.

Department of Employment, *Employment Protection Act 1978,* HMSO, London.

Department of Health, *The Health of the Nation 1992: A Strategy for Health in England,* HMSO, London.

Edwards, F.C., McCallum, R.I. *et al.* (1988) *Fitness for work – the medical aspects,* Oxford Medical Publications, Oxford.

HMSO (1974) *Health and Safety at Work Act 1974,* HMSO, London.

HMSO (1987) *Control of Substances Hazardous to Health Regulations 1988,* HMSO, London.

Health and Safety Executive, *Noise at Work Regulations 1989,* HMSO, London.

Health and Safety Executive, *Health and Safety (Display Screen Equipment) Regulations 1992,* HMSO, London.

Industrial Relations Series (IRS), Employment Trends 517, August 1992, IRS.

McEvoy, M., Porter, K. *et al.* (1987) Prospective study of clinical, laboratory and ancillary staff with accidental exposures to blood or body fluids from patients infected with HIV. *British Medical Journal,* **294**, 1585–7.

Raffle, Andrew (ed.) (1985) *Medical Aspects of Fitness to Drive – A Guide for Medical Practitioners,* (4th edn), Medical Commission on Accident Prevention, London.

Shaper, A.G., Cook, D.G. *et al.* (1984) Prevention of ischaemic heart disease in middle-aged British men. *British Heart Journal,* **51**, 595–605.

World Health Organisation (1992) Lifestyle and health risks at the workplace. *European Occupational Health Series,* **2**, WHO, Europe.

4

Work and change in industrial society: a sociological perspective

Andrew Cameron

INTRODUCTION: WHY IS WORK IMPORTANT?

Despite predictions of the 'collapse of work' or the arrival of the 'leisure society', it is clear that work continues to be a central institution in modern contemporary societies such as Britain.

The work that people do and how it is organized has profound consequences, both for society and for individuals. As well as economic rewards and wealth, work may provide identity and status as well as fulfilment and elation. Alternatively, stress, anxiety or boredom may be the outcome of work or, in the case of the unemployed, its absence. Health and relations with fellow human beings are influenced by work, as are patterns of leisure, family and community life. In consequence, the study of work can assist in the achievement of a fuller understanding of our own situation, as well as that of others.

Classical and contemporary sociologists have focused on many of the above facets of work, generating perspectives and empirical studies to enhance our understanding of work in industrial society. This chapter presents an overview of this work. It is intended to be intelligible both to those possessing a prior knowledge of sociology as well as those new to the subject. A selection of the sociological perspectives and themes on work in industrial society is provided and discussion of current trends in work, with particular reference to the UK.

The following three aspects of sociological enquiry are empha-sized and constitute a theme for the material presented:

- **Theories**: Theoretical perspectives, themes and issues which have influenced the way work is viewed and studied;
- **Facts and findings**: Selected empirical material on patterns of work and how it is changing in today's world;
- **Effects and consequences**: Practical implications of current and future trends in work, as they may affect both the indi-vidual and management.

SOCIOLOGICAL THEMES AND PERSPECTIVES ON WORK: ARE
THE 'OLD IDEAS' STILL RELEVANT?

The study of work was a central theme in the writings of the 'founding figures' of sociology. Although they wrote about 100 years ago, Karl Marx, Emile Durkheim and Max Weber identified issues which have been of continuing interest and influence on those with both academic and managerial interests.

Specialization and the division of labour

All three writers emphasized the significance of the increasing degree of specialization, or division of labour, associated with the coming of industrial society. The complex forms of work and their location in factories were contrasted with agrarianism and domestic systems of various pre-industrial societies.

The increasing division of labour was viewed in varying and contrasting ways by these early sociologists. In particular, the degree of optimism or pessimism attached to the consequences and implications of the division of labour and the response of workers to the form and shape of work in industrial society gave rise to differing views. In one sense, this new world of work was seen as presenting opportunities, as a break with the feudal and repressive past. Others saw a more foreboding world of 'dark satanic' factories and mills – one form of slavery replaced by another, equally or more repressive. A similar ambivalence exists today when questions are posed about the consequences of new technologies or major 'reorganizations' of work and their impact on employment, skill levels, job satisfaction and control.

Karl Marx: 1818–1883

Work and alienation

The idea that work is characterized by feelings of 'alienation' can be traced to the early writings of Marx and has subsequently become a recurring theme. The term alienation refers to the lack of power and unfulfilling character of labour when it is imposed and unsatisfying to the worker:

> How alien it really is is very evident from the fact that when there is no physical or other compulsion labour is avoided like the plague.
>
> (Marx, 1844)

Although it was in the nature of human beings to be creative and productive in their work, alienation, it was predicted, would be an increasingly widespread feature of work in capitalist society. It would cease only with the replacement of capitalism by a radically different form of society, where workers themselves owned and controlled the means of production.

Over a century later Robert Blauner's influential study (1967) reduced the concept of alienation to four dimensions of work. These were: powerlessness, meaninglessness, social isolation and self-estrangement.

	PRINTING	TEXTILES	MASS PRODUCTION	AUTOMATION
POWERLESSNESS	Low	High	High	Low
MEANINGLESSNESS	Low	High	High	Low
SOCIAL ISOLATION	Low	Low	High	Low
SELF-ESTRANGEMENT	Low	Low	High	Low

Blauner concluded from attitude surveys that the degree of alienation varied with the type of technology. As industrialism progressed from simpler technologies such as printing and textiles to mass production, alienation levels would rise. As industry entered the era of automation, Blauner, in contrast to Marx, predicted a move to lower levels of alienation at work (Blauner, 1967). For a summary and critical discussion of this study see Eldridge (1971).

Writers following the Marxist tradition (Braverman, 1974) have tended to reject Blauner's view that the problem of alienation can be overcome by technical reforms at work such as changes in job design, skill levels, or the adoption of more humanistic forms of management control. It would require the arrival of a form of 'post-capitalist' society, where work relations ceased to be exploitive, for work to cease to be alienating.

Work and class

A second theme in the Marxian perspective concerned the class-divided nature of capitalist societies. With respect to work, this 'social division of labour' emphasized unequal positions in the labour market. On one hand there were the manual workers, possessing little power and control over their work situation; on the other, owners of the means of production and those in élite occupational positions, exercising a high degree of control at work and receiving high rewards from it. It was predicted that such class division at work would broaden and polarize over time. Subsequently, evidence on the persistence of inequalities of pay, working conditions, health, gender, race and other features of work today have been cited, to argue that this view of a labour force divided along class lines still holds true.

As with 'alienation', Marxists see little prospect of a solution to these problems without a fundamental restructuring of society. Today, outside the Marxist tradition, there are various reformist approaches which advocate equal opportunities, profit-sharing, share ownership, enhanced working conditions and self-employment as answers to the issue of alienation and inequality at work. This reforming tradition stems from the work of functionalists such as Durkheim.

Emile Durkheim: 1858–1917

Work as community and co-operation

Much of the 'reforming' tradition is associated with Durkheim's 'functionalist' approach in sociology. In functionalist accounts and explanations, society is seen as an interrelated body, analogous to a biological system; each part of society is viewed in terms of its functional contribution to the rest of the system. Hence, in the case of work, functionalists stress the positive contributions work makes to society and the individual.

Durkheim (1984) viewed the extensive and increasing division of labour in a more positive or optimistic light than Marx. For Durkheim, work in industrial society was potentially functional, enabling the creation of a sense of interdependence between fellow workers. Work could be a source of social solidarity for the individual rather than disintegration. This theme of work as community was expected to be most pronounced among professional groups, leading to the formation of self-regulating 'occupational associations'. Subsequently, research has demonstrated the close ties that can exist between the workforce and the local community in mining villages and fishing communities. Human-relations theorists have established a tradition, following from the Hawthorne experiments, emphasizing the importance of work-group relations. The series of investigations conducted at the Hawthorne Plant of the Western Electric Company in Chicago drew attention to the importance of 'group norms' and informal relations in the workplace (Roethlisberger and Dickson, 1939; Rose, 1975). Many of today's ideas of team-working, quality circles and 'kaizen' associated with 'Japanization' follow this tradition.

Work as integration and individual identity

As well as creating a sense of solidarity, a further function of the extensive division of labour was to provide 'opportunities' for the wide range of individuals to develop their particular skills or capacities, or find their particular 'niche' in society. This was referred to as the 'spontaneous division of labour' with work facilitating a mobile, meritocratic or 'fluid' society.

Max Weber: 1864–1920

The work ethic: why do we work: cash or commitment?

Weber's general theory concerning the rationalization of life in industrial society stressed the importance of ideas or beliefs in providing a rationale for work. Work in capitalist society was underpinned by the religious views of Calvinism and the protestant ethic, associated with the reformation in Europe (Weber, 1991). In this view, work is seen as intrinsically good for its own sake; commitment to work, as a form of service or 'calling', goes beyond mere cash values. Such a belief about work continues to be encountered among some occupational groups today and has given rise to persistent debates about why people work, in particular, about the relative influences of pay and other factors in shaping work motivation and the perennial question of whether it is 'love or money' that draws people to work.

Bureaucracy: red tape or efficiency?

A further legacy from Weber stems from the theory of bureaucracy. Weber (1968) formulated an 'ideal type' model of bureaucracy which, he believed, despite its dehumanizing and oligarchic tendencies would become the blueprint for the organization of work in modern industrial societies. There have been widespread criticisms of bureaucracy and successive attempts to adapt and humanize the organization structures of modern business and administrative corporations. Nevertheless, the bureaucratic model and its companion – F.W. Taylor's (1911) *The Principles of Scientific Management* – continue to be the basis of most modern organizations today; the quest for 'alternative' or 'post-bureaucratic' structures is still an open issue in management literature (Clegg, 1990; Reed, 1992).

SUMMARY AND DISCUSSION

The purpose of the preceding section has not been to offer a history lesson cataloguing outmoded sociological ideas about the world of work but, rather, to show with selected examples that many of the issues pinpointed by the classical commentators still represent current debates about work today.

The classical themes and debates outlined:
• The division of labour and alienation
• Inequalities at work
• Work as a source of involvement and community
• Work as opportunity for personal advancement
• Work values and ideals
• Work organization and bureaucratic control

continue to be at the centre of much contemporary discussion and concern. A more extensive discussion of these classical 'strands of thought' can be found in Watson (1987). Among issues

absent from the classical agenda that have subsequently
attention are:

- the scale, extent and speed of technological changes at work
  and their impact upon health, attitudes and the quality of
  working life;
- the sexual division of labour with its emphasis on women in
  the labour process.

Two opposed theoretical models

The above assortment of themes and perspectives can be represented as two opposed general perspectives on work in industrial society. On the one hand a **Critical** view of work emphasizes the conflicts and alienating tendencies of work. On the other a **Functionalist** perspective, derived more closely from the work of Durkheim and Weber, emphasizes more positive aspects of work as a source of involvement, satisfaction and social solidarity.

The principal features of these contending ways of looking at work in industrial society are summarized below.

TWO PRINCIPAL PERSPECTIVES ON WORK IN INDUSTRIAL SOCIETY

FUNCTIONAL, CONSENSUS   CRITICAL, CONFLICT

MAJOR THEORISTS

Durkheim, Weber, Blauner   Marx, Braverman

MAIN FUNCTIONS AND FEATURES OF WORK

FUNCTIONAL, CONSENSUS	CRITICAL, CONFLICT
Source of individual identity	Alienating and unnatural
Economic rewards	Economic exploitation
Opportunity for advancement	Work a form of social control
Social co-operation and teamwork	Work divisive and competitive

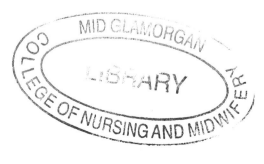

ROLE OF THE STATE

Employment legislation and industrial relations policies protect workers rights and provide framework for employee relations	Legislation and government policy favours employers
State as neutral 'referee'	State as representative of class interest

CURRENT AND FUTURE TRENDS

Technological progress leads to greater autonomy and increased skill levels	Technological changes lead to tighter control and reduced skill levels
Power at work becomes more widely distributed	Power concentrated in property-owning class or managerial élite
Quality of working life improves	Working life features new forms of deprivation and stress
Work tends to become source of social change and greater equality in society	Divisions in work persist and broaden
Work organization more flexible and post-bureaucratic	Organization continues to be hierarchical

WOMEN AND WORK

Greater participation, source of equality and role change	Gender divisions persist Women 'reserve pool of labour'

THE INDIVIDUAL AND WORK

Work less fragmented and specialized	New jobs frequently more fragmented and narrow than previous craft work
Trend towards more expressive attitudes	Work remains instrumental for majority

We now turn to examine a number of the principle trends and

changes occurring with respect to work and the division of labour.

THE CHANGING FACE OF WORK

The division of labour was identified earlier as a common theme in much of the thought and analysis of work. It can be broken down into a number of aspects:

1. **Occupational structure** – the general broad technical divisions of 'who does what' in society;

2. **The organization of work** – the specific arrangements whereby tasks are allocated and organized among groups of workers in the workplace;

3. **The individual** – focusing on the effects of work on peoples' attitudes, motivation and work behaviour.

In the following sections, the changes in these three aspects of the division of labour are summarized and the consequences and interpretations of these changes discussed in the light of the two contrasting perspectives outlined above.

Occupational structures

The principal UK trends and changes in occupational structure in recent years can be summarized as follows:

The shift from primary and secondary producing and manufacturing sectors, to tertiary or services;

The increase in white collar, professional and semiprofessional occupations, in contrast to blue collar manual work;

The increased participation of women in work and the decline in the activity rates of males;

The increase in the structural levels of unemployment;

Changes in union membership and industrial relations.

From primary producing to servicing: post-industrial society or business as usual?

The decline of agriculture and other primary producing over the last 150 years has been dramatic. In the middle of the nineteenth century around 22% of the UK workforce were employed in agriculture; today it is under 2%. The last two decades have witnessed a similar revolution in manufacturing employment. It fell from 36% in 1971 to a level of 22% in 1989. The tertiary or service sector, comprising a wide range of occupations from transport, retail trade, health and schools to banking and research has experienced a corresponding rise in numbers employed, from 55% to 69%.

One interpretation of the consequences of this change in occupational structure is that it indicates the arrival of a new kind of industrial order, a 'service' or 'post-industrial' society (Bell, 1973; Halmos, 1970; Gershuny, 1983). In particular, Daniel Bell's detailed portrait of post-industrialism envisages a society with the following features:

- Theoretical knowledge and expertise associated with service work replaces the labour power and traditional 'know-how' of manufacturing;
- A shift in power from the hands of the owners and controllers of the means of production into the hands of a managerial 'technocracy' comprising those with professional qualifications and expertise;
- The new managerialists, rewarded through salaries rather than profit, set different priorities or goals.

These new priorities and goals include:

- Long-term investment and development rather than short-term profit;
- Quality of service provided and customer satisfaction rather than material output;
- Enhanced levels of employee satisfaction and quality of working life in place of alienation and exploitation;
- In public corporations and government, social and cultural goals such as health, welfare and education replace economic ones.

Although in many respects plausible, this interpretation of changing occupational patterns has been questioned in a number of ways (Kumar, 1978; Crook *et al.*, 1992):

- Much of the new service sector has little to do with welfare and personal service. Frequently servicing the needs of manufacturing such as banking, transport, research and development, it remains profit and production orientated. Although the numbers employed directly in production have declined, the economy remains predominantly manufacturing- and output-dominated.
- Although many new managerialists owe their positions to technical expertise and qualifications, they frequently continue to be recruited from a narrow, élite band in society or become incorporated into the world of capital and profit by way of share ownership and profit-sharing.
- In the UK, public-sector cutbacks and a return to *laissez-faire* market principles has occurred, rather than the shift to welfare and cultural principles envisaged by Bell (1973). Various health-care occupations typify this change, where 'efficiency criteria' are frequently seen to be replacing patient care. In the UK, hospital 'trusts' and the 'local management of schools', like the privatized public corporations, are encouraged to operate on management systems where the balance-sheet takes precedence over the more personalized aspects of service.
- Although there is some evidence of changes in work practices towards an enhanced quality of working life, for the majority of workers even in the 'new' personal services such as health (Doyal, 1979) and catering (Gabriel, 1988), work remains hierarchically organized, routine, unfulfiling and insecure.

From blue collar to white collar: the decline of class at work?

Frequently, the shift from manufacturing to servicing is seen as synonymous with a growth of white collar work. This, in turn, is taken to symbolize the demise of the tall, triangular social structure, with sharply demarcated class divisions, associated with capitalism and emphasized in Marxist analysis. Instead, a flatter, diamond-shaped structure with an expanding middle-class, finer gradations between the strata, greater social mobility between the strata and less distance (in terms of pay differentials and working conditions) between the top and the bottom, characterizes the post-industrial society.

This view is consistent with Durkheim's vision of a fluid society and Weber's belief that the finer gradations of occupational status would replace the more rigid divisions of class as the basis of stratification in modern society. More recently, Dahrendorf (1959) has claimed that changes in work have, contrary to Marxist predictions, produced a fragmentation or decomposition of class. In Dahrendorf's model, not only the blurring of horizontal divisions of job status contribute to the break-up of class, but divisions within classes also contribute to reduced class solidarity. In all cases, technical changes in the division of labour or the 'jobs people do' are seen to be replacing social class as the bases of society's hierarchy. This view has been endorsed in recent years by those who maintain that we are now a 'postmodernist' society and that the link between work and political and class affiliation has been severed (Crook, Pakulski and Waters, 1992).

Others see the claim that the occupational shift from blue collar to white collar signifies a new social order as an exaggeration. The arguments against can be summarized as follows:

- Much of the new white collar work is middle-class only in name. Working in the fast-food industry, hospital cleaning or stacking supermarket shelves is only marginally different from the routine factory or blue collar work it replaced.
- Entry into occupations, particularly the more prestigious categories, is still largely 'class-based' and occupational and social mobility up and down the hierarchy is for the most part short-range (Goldthorpe *et al.*, 1987). Meteoric 'rags to riches' movements from the factory floor to the boardroom remain exceptional rather than commonplace.
- Inequalities in the rewards, outcomes and conditions of work still coincide with the broad class divisions of society. This includes the more obvious examples such as pay and fringe benefits, but other inequalities such as health, mortality and redundancy remain closely wedded to the status or category of work performed (Whitehead, 1987).

In the UK many of these inequalities associated with work have become accentuated during the past decade. In particular, it is widely acknowledged that the lower paid have seen a relative deterioration in their share of income during this period, as pay differentials have broadened. Between 1979 and 1991 the share of net pay received by the poorest fifth of the working population fell from 10% to 7%. Meanwhile, the highest paid fifth of the workforce extended their share by over 5%, from 35% to 41% (Social Trends, 1993). The removal of wages councils, which stipulate a minimum wage for workers in certain sectors, and resistance to European Union proposals for a minimum wage may lead to a continuation of this trend.

Professionalization: caring or controlling?

The phrase 'the professionalization of everyone' was coined more than 30 years ago to underline a trend occurring within the world of work. More jobs acquiring 'grand' titles, qualifications and training, as well as restrictions on entry, would characterize the more technocratic, or increasingly expert labour force of the future.

Recent figures for the UK categorize 35% of male workers and 28% of females, respectively, as 'managerial and professional'. This contrasts with a figure of just over 3% in 1921 and just under 11% in the 1971 census. The rise of professions is open to differing interpretations, signifying either the rise of caring, committed workers or the persistence of bastions of privilege and agents of control.

Despite this general rise in professional work, the 'élite professions' tend to have remained confined to a narrow range of privileged groups such as medicine and law. The main growth has taken place in a secondary strata of semi-professions, including teachers, nurses and paramedicals, social workers, accountants and estate agents. In certain cases it can be argued that occupational groups have experienced an element of de-professionalization. For example, the opthalmic opticians' monopoly over service provision has been eroded (Fielding, 1988); teachers have experienced a loss of autonomy and control over their work, and the traditional security and status of the clergy and public-sector professionals such as social workers and nurses has declined.

The model of the professions and the process of professionalization undertaken to acquire this status includes a number of the following traits or stages:

- Theoretical body of knowledge and training;
- Code of ethics and standards;
- Control over members;
- Collective culture or 'community';
- Autonomy.

The benefits accruing from an increasingly professionalized work-force are perhaps less clear-cut. Advantages such as:

- improved standards of training;
- availability of more and improved standards of expertise;
- professional commitment;
- complaints procedure for clients

need to be balanced against possible disadvantages of the professional model. From the client's viewpoint these include:

- restrictions on entry;
- perpetuation of élitism, inequality and privilege;
- poor communication with, and detachment from, clients;
- exploitation of power position regarding payment and the withholding of information from clients.

Blane (1991) discusses the strengths and weaknesses of the professional model with respect to health care and Illich (1975) provides a critical view in which the medical profession is described as a 'disabling profession'. The organization and provision of health care on the basis of the professional model and the resulting 'medicalization of health' mystifies health matters and undermines people's ability to know about and care for their own health. The professional health carer occupies a power position and may use language and high-technology methods in a way that alienates the patient. A similar position is explored by Abbot (1990) with respect to health visitors as agents of control.

Pilgrim and Rogers (1993) review the range of perspectives on professions, including:

- Durkheim's 'functional' or 'integrative' approach;
- Weber's 'self-interest' approach;
- Various Marxian debates about where professions stand in relation to ruling-class interests;
- Feminist perspectives, in which attention is drawn to the

variety of ways in which women are frequently subordinated by, and within, professions.

They follow this with a discussion of whether professions in the field of mental health serve as repressive agents of social control, labelling and crushing the individuality of those in their charge or, alternatively, whether they are a more benign force, committed to ameliorating the distress of their patients. More generally, Elston (1991) gives a detailed but inconclusive exploration of the ways in which medical professionals have been affected by recent reforms in the health service, in particular the rival arguments of 'proletarianization versus professionalization' in the face of the rise of the new breed of general managers.

The feminization of work: emancipation or exploitation?

The increased participation of married women in paid work outside the home represents one of the major recent changes in UK society.

Throughout the century the proportion of women who work has risen. Currently, 68% of women of working age work. With a corresponding drop in the activity rates for men, it is predicted that by the year 2000, women will account for more than 45% of the total labour force.

This changing status of women as workers is frequently interpreted as indicating the 'changing role of women in society', or the arrival of 'equality of the sexes'. The changes at work are seen as being reflected in the home, towards a pattern of equal 'role sharing', with spouses becoming partners at work and in the home. Willmott and Young (1973) predicted a trend towards the 'symmetrical family', where partners of both sexes would share equally in domestic and work roles. This process hinged largely on technical changes in the nature of work, leading to a breakdown in the sexual division of labour which traditionally saw masculinity being a necessary qualification for much blue collar manual work.

The culture of the workplace may also, in the future, reflect this change. Mills and Murgatroyd (1991) cite examples from North American studies where the values of competitiveness and aggression frequently associated with 'men's work in a man's world' and customarily found from the shop floor to the boardroom, can be challenged by collective action, corporate policy or the law. In the UK, entry to the medical profession appears to be more open to women; recruitment to medical schools currently includes just over 50% women, in contrast to the 35% of a decade ago (Doyal, 1979). These beliefs are reflected in policy initiatives such as the Equal Pay and Sex Discrimination Acts and, more recently, codes of practice relating to equal opportunities and sexual harassment. Although such measures are designed to recognize the position of women in the labour force and increase their representation in all sectors and levels of the workforce, 'the facts' remain unconvincing:

- Despite legislation, women's pay remains only around 60% –70% of that received by men for similar work;
- Women still perform 'women's work': 82% are in the service sector engaged in catering, secretarial, personal caring, cleaning and retail services. These work roles frequently service the needs of men, reinforcing the traditionally gendered or patriarchal nature of society.
- The persistence of a gender division at work is mirrored by its continuation in the home, where data from various studies suggest that the 'liberated' woman continues to perform a disproportionate share of domestic work (Gittins, 1982; General Household Survey, 1991). Studies of 'dual-working' couples emphasize stresses and role overload from the competing pressures of work and family life.
- More than 40% of women workers are part-time. They constitute the overwhelming majority of part-time workers; 7% are in temporary posts as against 4% of men. Part-time work may be attractive in some respects, but it carries with it many penalties, in particular lower pay, reduced job security and promotion prospects, fewer training and development opportunities and less holiday pay and other entitlements.
- The 'gendering' of work and the location of many women in a part-time labour market has been expressed as the 'dual labour market theory'. In this, women are a reserve pool of labour to be drawn on when the economy is growing and equally easily shed in times of recession.
- Finally, even where women succeed in entering traditionally male-dominated areas of work such as medicine and teaching they are likely to find themselves clustered in the lower ech-

elons and confronted by a variety of barriers increasing recognized as a 'glass ceiling'.

Decline in activity rates of males

The participation of men in the labour market has fallen in recent years from 90.4% in 1981 to 86.6% in 1990. This is accounted for by the decline in traditional manual blue collar employment sectors, giving rise to increased structural levels of unemployment and higher participation rates in education.

The shedding of labour from the traditional manufacturing and primary producing sectors has frequently been achieved through early retirement and voluntary redundancy. During the early 1980s this process tended to be viewed as a readjustment or 'shake-out' in the economy, with the hint that new jobs in the service or expanding industries would replace the traditional ones and unemployment would be 'frictional' and short-term rather than 'structural'. On the surface, this may seem to have a certain socially acceptable appeal, representing a timely and perhaps overdue demise in work which was often physically and psychologically damaging and afforded little job satisfaction. Against this has to be placed the adverse effects of enforced redundancy and long-term unemployment. Furthermore, many newly created jobs are in lower paid sectors, requiring less skill and offerring little meaning or job satisfaction. Finally, even the fear of unemployment increasingly figures as a cause of stress among those in work.

Unemployment: temporary 'blip' or permanent blight?

Despite policy initiatives such as redundancy counselling, job clubs, enterprise-allowance schemes, 'restart' interviews and employment training, little impact has been made on the underlying trend towards male and female worklessness. Unemployment rates for men and women, in Britain, have followed similar general patterns over the last two decades. From just under 4% in 1971, unemployment for men rose steadily to a peak of 13% in 1986; the fall to 8% in 1989 was followed by a sharp rise to 12% in 1992. In 1993 the total number of unemployed came close to the 1986 peak of over three million and the core of long-term unemployed (one year or more without work) continues to move towards the one million mark. There would seem little prospect of a return to the 'full employment' of the 1960s. Writers such as Atkinson (1988) view this as a new and perhaps permanent state, where the labour market will continue to feature a pool of both short-term and long-term unemployed.

Within these broad trends, unemployment follows varying patterns according to factors such as gender, age, ethnicity and region:

- Although the official rates for women are lower than for men – 7.2% compared with the 11.5% in 1992 (*Social Trends*, 1993) – they almost certainly understate the picture, as the incentive for many women to register is reduced by the benefits' system. Similarly, the likelihood of women experiencing the loss of their job is greatly increased by their position in the 'reserve pool of labour';
- Workers aged 50 and over are more likely to lose their job; this often means they are unlikely to work again. The trend to such forced early retirement has implications for the ageing process as well as the health and welfare of the older members of society;
- Youth unemployment is particularly acute. In 1989 the rate for under–25-year-olds was a little under 10%, against approximately 6% for the population as a whole. Youth-training schemes make it difficult to obtain a true figure for young people under 18 seeking work;
- Among men, manual workers are more likely to lose their jobs than their non-manual counterparts and unskilled manual workers are three times more likely to be hit by unemployment than average;
- Black and Asian workers have higher rates. For Afro-Carribean males, rates are twice that for white workers and for Pakistani/Bangladeshis nearly 3 times higher. This is partly attributable to discrimination and also skill levels;
- Marked regional differences exist. In 1990 the South East and East Anglia had less than 4% unemployed while Scotland and Northern Ireland were over 12%. Inner-city areas have male rates over 20%, whilst some 'shire' areas have less than 3%.

Apart from the obvious economic consequences, there is growing evidence that long-term unemployment has a range of social and psychological effects. Jahoda's (1982) study pinpointed the sense of purposelessness that results from destruction of domestic routine, a view supported by more recent evidence in a collection of studies by Gallie *et al.* (1994). Portwood (1985) similarly identified social isolation and fatalistic resignation. Various studies such as Knox *et al.* (1985) indicate that unemployment contributes to high blood pressure and increased heart disease among the unemployed. Jacobson, Smith and Whitehead (1991) quote evidence that death rates for unemployed men and their wives are 20% higher than expected and suicide rates are double those of the employed. Whitehead (1987) quotes various studies on unemployment and attempted suicide. These indicate that the rate increases with the duration of unemployment: those who have been out of work for more than 12 months have rates 19 times greater than their employed counterparts. Greater incidence of marriage breakdown and mental health complete the toll of effects.

These trends and patterns emphasize the structural and political nature of unemployment, that it is a 'price to pay' in the battle against inflation. This effectively undermines the case that unemployment is an individual phenomenon 'caused' by lazy people not wishing to work – a popular notion encouraged by frequent mass-media references to 'scroungers'. Nevertheless, much of the policy and measures aimed at reducing unemployment focus on individuals, encouraging them to seek work and find their own solutions to the problem. This is often demeaning and introduces an element of 'victim-blaming' into a situation which requires structural changes and economic regeneration. Among suggestions aimed at producing longer term structural responses to unemployment are: investment in new jobs in the service sector, shorter working hours, job-sharing, part-time work and re-training. Nevertheless, there seems little evidence that a return to the full employment of the 1960s is other than a remote possibility which would suggest the need to concentrate more resources on reducing the effects of unemployment and its human cost.

Trades unions and industrial conflict: new realism or union bashing?

A final area of change in the general 'contours of work' in contemporary Britain revolves around the debate about the changing patterns of trades-union activity and employee relations. One popular interpretation is that the various changes in membership and union activity indicate the arrival of a new realism in industrial relations and a shift from a world in which work, for many, signified social solidarity and class action to one of *laissez-faire* and individualism.

The principal changes associated with this transformation have been relatively long-term trends which have become accentuated in Britain during the 1980s and 1990s and are particularly associated with the era of Thatcherism. They comprise the following:

- Decline in trades-union membership, particularly in 'traditional blue collar' sectors. The period 1979 to 1990 saw a 25% fall in membership;
- Decline in strikes and numbers of days lost through industrial action to record low levels;
- A reduction in the number of different trades unions as a result of mergers.

More specific to the late 1980s are: a move towards single union or 'company' agreements, where an employer chooses to recognize just one union to represent the whole of the workforce, rather than granting negotiating rights to a range of different unions according to trade, skill or profession.

In some cases such 'single table' agreements, negotiated by firms and some hospital trusts, have been accompanied by procedural arrangements amounting to 'no strike deals'. Similarly, in some instances, employers have 'de-recognized' unions, choosing to negotiate directly with the labour force as individuals or through the medium of works' councils or staff associations.

The 1980s also saw an unprecedented succession of legislative measures aimed at reforming industrial relations. These changes in the law were a central feature of conservative government legislation built on the frequently voiced view that the unions had become too powerful. Poor labour relations, restrictive practices and stoppages at work, it was believed, were largely responsible for Britain's relative industrial decline and poor economic performance.

The main impact of the legislation has been to reduce the power of the unions to take strike action, by insisting on strike ballots and making secondary picketing illegal. Unofficial strikes have effectively been outlawed, as has the closed shop. Coupled with a tightening up of the legislation relating to unfair dismissals, these changes have been taken to symbolize a fundamental shift from 'voluntarism' to more legalistic forms of industrial relations. Similarly, a shift in power has favoured management, restoring the 'right to manage'. Supporters of these reforms in labour relations see them as giving unions back to their members, introducing democratic measures through strike ballots and curbing what were seen as the excessive powers of unions over their members.

This 'new realism' in employee relations is viewed by supporters as heralding a new era of freedom from strikes and co-operation in industry, to enhance the competitiveness and efficiency of British industry. Traditional 'working-class collectivism and solidarity' is viewed as outmoded, as employers increasingly choose to deal directly with employees rather than via the unions. More individualistic ideologies and approaches to work and its rewards are seen as being consistent with work in a postmodern or post-industrial context.

Alternatively, those who support the traditional rights of trades unions to act on behalf of their members view this period of 'union bashing' as signifying the destruction of the three-way consensus between employees, government and unions which characterized the earlier period of the 1960s and 1970s. This form of corporatism, where economic planning and wages policy were sought by way of consensus, conciliation and voluntary agreements, is seen as preferable to confrontation and legal measures, as used in the mining, printing and steel disputes. The 'collective' approaches, favoured in Japan, Germany and Scandinavia, are still seen to be applicable and the British return to confrontational policies in employee relations is seen as retrograde. The record low rates of strikes and industrial action result not from legislative reforms and the new realism, so much as from the record levels of unemployment which have characterized much of the 1980s. Similarly, the erosion of collective and solidaristic approaches to employee relations, and the increasing use of individual contracts of employment and performance-related pay systems, are viewed negatively. It is believed that such measures will create an atmosphere of 'divide and rule' among the workforce, facilitating the extension of divisions and inequalities among employees, particularly those sections with low skills or bargaining power. The view favoured by the government, that employee relations and management systems of the private sector can be effectively deployed in the public sector, is open to question. Storey (1992) argues that in the health service various political and organizational constraints work against such a transfer and that the professional orientation and commitment to patient care calls for the continuation of more 'collegiate' approaches.

Summary

Fundamental changes are occurring in the broad contours of occupational structure or division of labour in the UK. These changes are widely believed to influence many aspects of life in Britain today. What is less clear is the precise nature of these effects. In keeping with the two perspectives outlined in the introduction, the evidence can be viewed on the one hand as heralding a new, cleaner, technologically more efficient world of work where more people can participate in a climate of increased equal opportunities and harmonious labour relations. Alternatively, the collapse of traditional manufacturing is seen by others to signify new structures and old problems. Less skilled and lower paid service-sector work and increased levels of unemployment bring about a division of labour where large numbers of the labour force are relegated to 'periphery', featuring little security and promotion opportunities, low levels of pay and few prospects of achieving identity and fulfilment through work.

THE ORGANIZATION OF WORK

A second level of analysis of the division of labour centres on the organization of work. For most people work is conducted within the confines and pressures of some kind of organization, be it large, small, profit-making or voluntary. This aspect of work has attracted a great deal of attention from both academics and managers and is recognized as a field of study in its own right, usually referred to as 'organization theory' or 'organization analysis'. In general, the aims of organization theory have entailed identifying organization structures which engender success and efficiency at work.

In the same way that occupational structure is undergoing fundamental changes, so, it is frequently argued, organizations are taking on new forms in the modern world. The traditional, classical approaches based on the rigid, dogmatic principles predicted by Weber are being replaced by more flexible, varied structures. This possible trend in organization structures may be viewed by tracing the development of various approaches or perspectives in organization theory. Three approaches to organization structure with their respective strengths and weaknesses tend to have dominated the literature:

• Classical and scientific management approaches;
• Human-relations approaches;
• Systems and contingency approaches.

Contemporary ideas, frequently entitled human resource-management approaches and labelled 'new', 'postmodernist' or 'post-bureaucratic' tend to be new syntheses drawn from the earlier repertoire of ideas.

Classical approaches: the organization as a 'machine'

The classical approaches are associated with Max Weber's ideal type model of bureaucracy and Frederick Taylor's 'scientific management', the latter based on practical studies in the steel industry. Together they advocate organization structures containing the following features:

• **Specialized** and demarcated roles within the organization;
• **Hierarchical** systems of authority and control.

In addition, the smooth running of the organization is to be guaranteed by a set of:

• **Impersonal rules** and procedures covering every aspect of the organization's conduct.

These rules are to be rooted in 'rational principles' thereby ensuring the:

• **Individual freedom** of employees and subordinates.

The criticisms and limitations of these models have been well-documented and include the following:

• The 'machine like' nature, with its tendency to reduce people to 'mere cogs in a machine', has led to criticisms that the classical models are inhuman. In failing to recognize the social and psychological needs, the informal relationships and creative strengths of people at work, such structures become both alienating and inefficient. Subsequently, human-relations theorists have advocated forms of work organization where individuals perform a wider range of less specialized tasks, organized around the work group rather than the individual.

- Bureaucratic structures in many instances may be 'dysfunctional', producing the reverse of what was planned. 'Goal displacement', a process whereby the organization loses sight of its original purpose or substitutes some alternative goal, has been used to label this process. Similarly, groups or individuals may pursue sectional interests in opposition to other departments. These and other shortcomings are frequently voiced by those claiming bitter experience, such as 'one hand of the organization not knowing what the other is doing'. Or the cry of 'too much red tape', indicating the inability of the classical organization to change or respond quickly to a new situation because of its tall, hierarchical communication structures and its intricate system of rules.

- The potential for over-centralized control, abuse of power and 'oligarchy' in general resides in the hierarchical nature of classical command structures. More recent management ideologies frequently make the case for participative rather than autocratic styles of leadership and control, in the belief that these can be more efficient and motivating for subordinates.

- Finally, the universalistic claims of the classical models, advocating the same basic principles and structures for all organizations, regardless of their specific goals, technologies, or other contextual factors, have been refuted. In particular, 'contingency theorists' advocate a 'horses for courses' approach, whereby organizational structures and systems are tailored to the specific characteristics of the individual organization in question.

Despite these widespread criticisms of work organization, the classical models have remained resilient to change. For most people, work continues to be specialized and fragmented and is conducted in an environment of inflexible rules and hierarchical 'top-down' control systems. Morgan (1991) outlines the persistence of such hierarchical models in hospitals and some of the conflicts and tensions this produces in pursuing the multiple goals of such organizations.

The two principal departures from the dominant classical view have been, first, those derived from human relations perspectives and second, the contingency model, derived from open systems theories.

Human-relations approaches: organizations as people

The human-relations perspective arose as a criticism of the anti-humanistic aspects of the classical model summarized above. Following pioneering work by Elton Mayo in interpreting the famous Hawthorne studies and subsequent developments by Argyris (1964), Likert (1961), McGregor (1960) and Herzberg, Mansuer and Snyderman (1959), a perspective arose in which the workplace is seen as a social situation with informal structures and relationships. Human-relations theorists believe that people, by nature, wish to be involved and creative in their work situation and that appropriate structures and strategies can engender higher levels of commitment and motivation, thereby achieving the dual goal of raised output and a less alienated workforce. The principle practical measures advocated to facilitate improved integration of the individual and the organization are:

- Group and team structures;
- Participative and supportive styles of management, leadership and communication;
- 'Enriched' job design based less on specialization and more on job satisfaction.

Likert's overlapping group structure illustrates what such structures might look like in practice. In contrast to the 'line and staff' advocated in traditional models, the structure is seen as consisting of a number of overlapping groups co-ordinated by 'link pins'. As well as uniting a number of the human-relations principles, it anticipated many of the more recent ideas about flexibility and teamwork associated with Japanization.

There are a number of examples of organizations attempting to restructure according to such principles. ICI's job-enrichment programme and the so-called Volvo experiment (Berggren, 1993) are among the best known.

Such practices have not been widely implemented by management in the past. Trades unions and workers tended to be mistrustful, seeing such changes as potentially manipulative, while management appeared unimpressed by the productivity gains or the commitment to make it work in their particular industry. An additional reservation about these approaches gained strength in the UK with the publication of research (Goldthorpe *et al.*, 1968) which emphasized the problems of over-generalizing about what individuals require from work. They drew particular attention to the existence of complex variations existing in individuals' orientations to work and found that instrumentalism or 'cash rewards' were emphasized by workers, rather than the 'expressive' or self-actualizing needs emphasized in the human-relations model.

Systems and contingency approaches: organizations as 'biological organisms'

These approaches combine ideas from the classical and human-relations perspectives. Work is seen as consisting of a technical dimension requiring an element of concrete structure but also a social aspect, placing pressure on the organization to be flexible and humanistic. The systems view of work organization also contributed to a change in organizational perceptions or 'images', departing from the rigid fixed views of organizations to a view containing the following elements:

- **Organic analogy**: the organization is viewed as flexible and dynamic, akin to a living body, rather than being a rigid, machine-like entity;
- **Differentiated structures**: the organization is viewed as being made up of 'sub-systems', functionally interrelated like the organs of a body, each giving to and taking from the whole;
- **Environmental equilibrium**: to survive, the organization needs to adapt to environmental changes including such factors as competition, technical developments, social, demographic and political changes.

Although the biological analogy may seem strained, many people view organizations in such a way, frequently talking of healthy organizations, capable of development and growth. The systems perspective underpins many contemporary management-development and organizational-change programmes. The major advance to emerge from the systems perspective was the emphasis on the environment and the requirement that organizations be viewed as in a constant state of change and dynamic equilibrium or 'homeostasis' with their environment. This more flexible view of organizations also encouraged the development of contingency approaches. These identified a wider repertoire of possible organizational forms to be applied in different situations.

In rejecting the 'one best way' approach, they argued that the answer to choosing an appropriate organizational design lay in detailed consideration of a range of factors. Of these, some were internal, such as organizational size and type of work, but others, such as rate of technological change and external economic factors, lay outside the factory gate or office block.

Burns and Stalker (1961) provided one of the clearest original examples of such a contingency approach. Following detailed empirical studies of management in a number of companies they put forward the idea that there existed alternative ways of organizing. At one extreme were 'mechanistic' approaches, broadly similar to the 'bureaucratic' approach outlined above; on the other hand 'organic' structures were much closer to the flexible and humanistic approaches advocated by human-relations theorists.

Organic structures featured:

- Contributive nature of specialization, and realistically defined tasks;
- Continual redefinition of tasks through interaction and flexible definition of rights and obligations;
- Network and lateral structure of communications, control and consultation;
- Commitment to the overall task of the organization with high value placed on knowledge of the world outside the organization.

Put simply, Burns and Stalker's message that there is 'no one best way' to organize advocated a contingency model as follows:

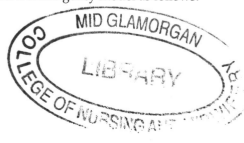

	STRUCTURE		ENVIRONMENT
MECHANISTIC STRUCTURES	— appropriate in —	STABLE ENVIRONMENTS
ORGANIC STRUCTURES	— appropriate in —	UNSTABLE ENVIRONMENTS

Environmental stability reflected such things as the rate of technological change, competition and government policy. Today, an illustration of the need for organizations to respond to environmental considerations in planning and structuring can be seen from Britain's membership of the EC single market. As well as the commercial implications EC regulations on matters such as working conditions and health and safety regulations, they have significant implications for UK organizations and their human-resource management strategies.

Recent restructuring in the health, education and public utilities sectors towards greater market orientation and competitiveness is also a form of response to external environmental influences. The adoption of local management of schools, hospital-trust status, community-care policies and contracting out in the public sector illustrates the magnitude of organizational change influencing work organization today. These examples underline the importance of looking at factors outside the organization in understanding people's work today.

CONTEMPORARY TRENDS IN THE ORGANIZATION OF WORK: NEW WINE IN OLD BOTTLES?

Recent examples of organizational change and restructuring consistent with some aspects of the trend towards more organic and humanistic form of organizational structure are Japanization and the flexible organization.

Japanization

Japanization describes the process of transferring elements of the Japanese corporate form of work organization, with its distinct cultural and economic features, to other societies and cultures, such as the UK and the US.

The main features of the Japanese system include the following:

- Lifetime commitment/job for life;
- Familial structure and relationships;
- Collective (as opposed to individualistic) orientation;
- Promotion and remuneration on the basis of seniority;
- Company welfare schemes;
- 'Single' or company unions.

In addition, a number of techniques associated with the organization and control of work are frequently featured in such systems, for example:

- Kanban or 'just in time' production control;
- Kaizen: group-based critical-analysis techniques;
- Quality-management systems;

The origins, transferability and persistence of Japanization are subject to discussion. From a managerial perspective it is frequently represented as a form of work organization with the capacity to redress Britain's problem of low productivity and economic decline. The advantages of team-working and a more corporate culture of togetherness, with fewer of the 'us and them' cleavages associated with UK industry, plus the higher levels of commitment and motivation, are frequently emphasized. Alternatively, more critical sociological perspectives tend to be reserved and sceptical. The overarching success of Japanese corporatism is questioned. It accounts for only 30% of Japanese production and is supported by a large 'secondary' labour market of insecure, part-time female labour, brandishing few of the benefits of the 'Japanese system'. The paternalism is seen as a return to employer-dominated labour relations, the teamworking as a reworking of old and frequently discredited human-relations techniques. A recent study of Japanization in the north east of England (Garrahan, 1992) emphasizes this other side. The study shows how the large corporation, located in an area of high unemployment and economic decline, may dominate aspects of the local culture and indoctrinate the workforce. The paradox whereby togetherness and collective teamworking is underpinned by strongly individualistic systems of appraisal and payment, reminiscent of Taylorism, is emphasized. This reinforces the view that, while organizations may have collective, interactive and participative working methods, the basic control methods remain hierarchical and formalized.

The flexible organization

The notion of flexible control, like Japanization, came to symbolize a new approach to organizing work in the late 1980s. Flexibility includes two particular aspects:

- Functional flexibility, entailing working methods and practices whereby workers would be multi-skilled and expected to perform a range of different skills and tasks, thereby reversing the ideology of rigid specialization and demarcation which was often portrayed as bedevilling British industry;
- Numerical flexibility where the labour supply comprises a core of skilled permanent workers supplemented by a reserve pool or 'periphery' of part-timers, sub-contractors, homeowrkers and the self-employed. The organization is thus enabled to respond more effectively to fluctuations in demand for goods or services.

The appeal of such flexible organization to management is easy to understand and consistent with the organic systems mentioned above. From a more critical perspective it can be seen why, in some circumstances, workers may be less than enthusiastic.

The 'opened-ended' nature of job descriptions in flexible organizations, whereby employees can be expected to perform any duty they are called upon to do, can be seen as threatening. It may well undermine the workers' autonomy and sense of expertise or professionalism. Taken to its logical conclusion such a 'jack of all trades' approach can bring erosion of skill levels for the employee and reduced levels of expertise. It often means that although 'qualified' and expected to perform a range of tasks, the opportunity to become competent and trained in a wide range of skills is not always provided. Stress and health and safety issues may arise when workers are obliged to carry out work for which they are unsuited or inadequately trained.

Similarly, being part of a 'flexible' secondary or peripheral labour force – a fate shared by an increasing proportion of the labour force – is not a universally attractive proposition. Workers in this sector frequently find themselves disadvantaged in a number of respects:

- Lower rates of pay;
- Fewer statutory rights, such as sick leave and employment protection;

- Fewer fringe benefits, such as holiday pay, pensions, staff development and training;
- Fewer opportunities for promotion.

Postmodern organizations

The team-working and flexibility outlined in the two preceding sections are frequently associated with a new era of 'postmodern' organization (Clegg, 1990; Reed, 1992). The postmodern organization typically includes the following structural features:

- A shift away from large-scale mass-production methods and products;
- Increased emphasis on consumer choice, responsiveness and quality of products and services;
- Greater individuality and self-actualization among 'core' workers;
- Increased decentralization of the organization's activities, including 'networking', sub-contracting, franchizing and collaboration between organizations.

Recently Fox (1993) vividly illustrated the application of a postmodern perspective as a way of looking at organizational life on the ward round in a hospital. In this account the fixed, rigid and objective aspects of organizational reality are seen to count less than the flexibility and negotiation used by the more powerful – in this case the surgeons – to impose their definition of organizational reality on the patients in their care. The ritual of the ward round, the language employed and the white coats of the staff are used as ways of minimizing the questions and threats to the wisdom and power of the medical staff. The study effectively echoes the influential notion of hospitals as 'total institutions' made famous by Goffman (1961) more than thirty years ago.

Summary

The way in which work is organized for many people today is certainly undergoing extensive change, with few public or private-sector organizations not experiencing some form of major reorganization. Organization theory presents a repertoire of approaches to such a problem, ranging from the rigid and machine-like bureaucratic structures of the classical schools, to the more people-centered, flexible and humanistic approaches advocated by human-relations theorists and some more recent exponents of modern human-resource management. Increasingly, these trends are seen as constituting a 'sea change' in organizational forms, earning the label 'postmodern' or 'post-bureaucratic'. What is less clear is whether the modern organizational rhetoric of flexibility, empowerment, worker autonomy and teamwork represents genuine basic changes in the principles and practice of modern organization, or whether it is superficial 'add ons' on structures that still remain at heart centralized, impersonal and manipulative.

WORK AND THE INDIVIDUAL: ATTITUDES TO WORK

The third aspect of work deals with the individual's views and feelings about the nature and organization of their work. In particular: what are the various factors influencing attitudes to work? In what ways are work attitudes changing, as a result of the structural and organizational factors listed above?

A frequent line taken in answering these two linked questions draws heavily on Maslow's 'hierarchy of needs' (1957) and Herzberg, Mausner and Snyderman's (1959) two-factor theory of work motivation. The explanation adopts the following logic:

1. Individuals have a range of personal, psychological and social needs. They seek 'self-actualization' and satisfaction of these needs at work;
2. As individuals achieve increased fulfilment of the 'higher order' needs of ego-involvement and self-actualisation at work, so their levels of job satisfaction and motivation will rise;
3. Technological advances enable the worst kinds of poorly paid, physically and mentally damaging work to be automated out and replaced by more skilled work. Increased skill levels provide opportunities for greater self-actualization.
4. Technological change is accompanied by management adopting more humanistic and flexible organizational cultures and management styles, redesigning and 'enriching' jobs to make them more intrinsically satisfying and improving the climate of human relations.
5. The resulting increased levels of commitment and greater

efficiency at work provide opportunities for further technological development and investment in human capital.

The above line of argument constitutes the ideology underpinning many modern human-resource strategies including the
following:

- Sophisticated job design and recruitment techniques;
- Commitment to technical training and employee devel-
  opment;
- Open channels of communication, such as the 'cascade'
  system;
- Job enrichment;
- Flexi-time, job-sharing, equal-opportunities commitments;
- Collaborative and team structures;
- 'Empowerment' of workforce.

Is it that simple?

Other writers express reservations about the above beliefs and
practices:

- The assumption that all people seek to satisfy a similar range
  of needs through their work has been questioned. Sociologists,
  particularly those writing from a phenomenological or relativ-
  ist perspective (Silverman, 1970; Rose, 1975; Morgan, 1986)
  stress the unique, wide-ranging different meanings and expectations individuals bring to their work. These may arise from
  variations in individual or psychological characteristics, or
  from different orientations, rooted in culture, age, gender
  or educational experiences. Furthermore, they may alter over
  time, or from one situation to another.
- Similarly, the idea that individuals will react or respond to
  work design or 'enlightened' management styles in a predi-
  cable or standard way is open to question. Changes at work,
  however benevolent or well-intended, are frequently resisted
  or treated with hostility or cynicism by the work force.
- Third, empirical studies show that workers frequently shun
  job improvement or enrichment programmes designed to
  make their work more varied or motivating, preferring instead
  to take an instrumental or economic view of their work, seeking self-actualization outside it.

- Those who follow Braverman's (1974) 'deskilling' or degradation of work theme take issue with the thesis that technological progress will, as a matter of course, produce jobs of a more intrinsically satisfying and less onerous nature. For these writers, the recent history of automation and technological advance is, rather, one of undermining skill levels and the autonomy of the craft worker. While some new skills may be developed as a result of technical development, losers as well as winners result from this process and the 'deskilling' versus 'enskilling' debate remains an open question.
- Lastly, there is an increasing awareness that while 'new jobs' may lack the physical deprivations and hardships of underground mining, deep-sea fishing, foundry or dock work they may still be characterized by boredom, high stress levels, repetitive strain or other harmful effects, such as the 'sick building syndrome'.

Other relevant factors

The 'motivation question' remains a complex issue and there has been a growing awareness that simple answers and explanations are unacceptable. In trying to comprehend our own feelings towards work or those of others, it is now clear that a wide range of factors need to be taken into account. These can be summarized as follows:

1. **Intrinsic** to the job, comprising:
   - technical aspects of the job;
   - skill levels;
   - responsibilities;
   - variety and range of tasks.
2. **Extrinsic** to the job. Although features of the workplace, these factors are not part of the job itself. These are increasingly referred to as organizational 'culture' or 'climate':
   - relationships with fellow workers;
   - supervision and management style;
   - pay and rewards;
   - working conditions and environment;
   - company policy.
3. **External or Extra Organizational**. These are external to the workplace. Together they influence the expectations and orien-

tations which people bring to work. They constitute the individual actors 'frame of reference':
- individual skill differences and perceptions;
- previous work experiences;
- cultural and traditional expectations;
- social class factors;
- gender;
- family and community influences;
- labour market factors;
- political and ideological factors.

Typical orientations

The predisposed views and expectations that individuals bring to the work situation, in contrast to those aspects of behaviour that may be conditioned by the work itself, are referred to as 'orientations'. Typical 'orientations' arising from the individual's links with the wider society have been labelled as follows:

- **Solidaristic**: traditional blue collar orientation emphasizing close relationships with fellow workers, tightly knit communities and predisposition to collective trades-union solidarity. Intrinsic rewards may be low, such as in coal mining and some uniformed services.
- **Professional**: emphasizing long-term commitment to career and service provision, high intrinsic job rewards such as in medicine, law and teaching.
- **Bureaucratic**: emphasis on loyalty, career and service to employer. High extrinsic job rewards such as fringe benefits and job security may be 'tied' to one employer, such as in clerks, semi-professionals such as local government officers and banking staff.
- **Instrumental**: little attachment to job, employer or fellow workers, main emphasis on cash and other extrinsic rewards, such as in an assembly-line worker.

'Fitting' individuals and jobs: is there a pattern?

Among the varying orientations and views of work, a contrast is frequently made between instrumental or cash orientations in contrast to expressive or 'self-actualizing'. It is possible to present a rudimentary contingency model where the individual worker's generalized orientation is related to job content and other aspects of the work situation. In this it can be argued that individuals with expressive or self-actualizing needs are more likely to exhibit positive attitudes and levels of motivation where the job is challenging. Alternatively, individuals with a more predominantly instrumental disposition to work are more likely to report satisfaction where the job is relatively routine and unchallenging.

Such a perspective on the individual and work question has a number of implications for human resource-management policies such as recruitment, training and job design. Modern corporations, in addition to the aptitude and personality testing traditionally associated with recruitment processes, are now paying increasing attention to matching the individual's disposition to the organization culture.

While in one sense the implication that people may be 'fitted' to jobs – some being 'screened out' altogether – has a somewhat manipulative and ethically unacceptable ring to it, the recognition that both individuals and job factors vary and may be matched in a variety of combinations and ways opens up certain more optimistic possibilities. Increasingly there would seem to be no logical reason why an era in which jobs might be fitted to people, rather than vice versa, may not ensue. Technological change is an important enabling factor and certain trends associated with new patterns of work by writers such as Handy (1984) include:

- flexible working hours;
- home-based working;
- job-sharing;
- 'portfolio working' (a number of different jobs held at once);
- job design to afford equal opportunities to disabled people;
- career breaks

and the optimistic suggestion that there may be increasing room to achieve an improved balance between an individual's needs and their work commitments.

CONCLUSION

A number of the principal changes occurring in the world of work today have been reviewed in this chapter. They have been discussed under the three headings of:

- occupational structure;
- work organization; and
- work and the individual.

The changes have been examined against a background of the differing sociological traditions developed in this area and particular stress has been placed on the contrasting ways in which changes and trends may be interpreted – an optimistic interpretation as against a less enthusiastic view of the future of work. In many cases such changes are, in essence, continuations of the technical and social changes in the division of labour outlined by the writers summarized in the early part of the chapter. Similarly the 'problem' of organization exposed by Weber – how to combine efficiency with humanistic organization – like the alienation theme continues to be a feature of contemporary concern. Although work is changing rapidly in many respects, the view offered in this chapter is that it will continue, at least for the foreseeable future, to be a fundamentally important social institution and process. Furthermore, the 'problems' and 'issues' – both theoretical and practical – that surround work will remain for the most part consistent with those 'traditional' ones raised by the classical writers.

As to the more recent trends in work discussed above including white collar service work, women working, flexible, 'postmodern' organization and new technology and motivational patterns, it does seem to be the case that the ambivalent optimistic or pessimistic interpretations remain applicable with respect to these as well, there being no single 'right' or 'wrong' answers to these important issues. Thus, for many, the shift towards non-union organized, home-based, flexi-working may appear as a form of 'postmodernist' liberation of a de-alienating and post-bureaucratic nature. For others, the prospect of part-time working in the periphery of the labour market, with minimal security and predictability and basic working conditions, may seem a foreboding or retrograde step.

Thinking and analysing the world of work from these alternating perspectives has, it is hoped, a twofold value. First, we may understand our own position, prospects, aspirations and frustrations in the labour market more clearly, thus being better prepared and empowered to come to terms with our own situation and the inevitable changes likely to confront us as members of the workforce. Second, if we work, as increasing numbers do, in servicing or managing the health, welfare and personal needs of others, it is important to have an understanding of the client's world of work. In many instances, effective and satisfactory performance of our own work roles may well hinge on having such an understanding of those we serve. Unemployment, stress, work-related diseases as well as the more routine organizational aspects of work leave their mark on people. To ignore this is to deny ourselves valuable insights into the live of others.

REFERENCES AND FURTHER READING

Abbott, P. (1990) Health visitors: policing the family, in Abbott, P. and Wallace, C. *The Sociology of the Caring Professions*, The Falmer Press, London.

Allen, S. *et al.* (1986) *The Experience of Unemployment*, Macmillan, Basingstoke.

Argyris, C. (1964) *Integrating the Individual and the Organisation*, Wiley, New York.

Atkinson, J. (1988) Recent changes in the internal labour market structure in the UK, in Buitelaar, W. (ed.) *Technology and Work: Labour Studies in England, Germany and The Netherlands*, Avebury, Aldershot.

Bell, D. (1973) *The Coming of Post Industrial Society*, Basic Books, New York.

Berggren, C. (1993) *The Volvo Experience*, Macmillan, Basingstoke.

Blane, D. (1991) Health professionals, in Scambler, G. (ed.) *Sociology as Applied to Medicine*, Bailliere Tindall, London.

Blauner, R. (1967) *Alienation and Freedom*, Chicago Press, Chicago.

Braverman, H. (1974) *Labour and Monopoly Capitalism: The Degradation of Work in the Twentieth Century*, Monthly Review Press, New York.

Burns, T. and Stalker, G.M. (1961) *The Management of Innovation*, Tavistock, London.

Clegg, S.R. (1990) *Modern Organisations: Organisation Studies in the Post Modern World*, Sage, London.

Crook, S., Pakulski, J. and Waters, M. (1992) *Postmodernization: Change in Advanced Society*, Sage, London.

Dahrendorf, R. (1959) *Class and Class Conflict in Industrial Society*, Routledge, Kegan & Paul, London.

Doyal, L. (1979) *The Political Economy of Health*, Pluto, London.

Durkheim, E. (1984) *The Division of Labour in Society*, Macmillan, Basingstoke.

Eldridge, J.E.T. (1971) *Sociology and Industrial Life*, Nelson, London.

Elston, M. (1991) The politics of professional power: medicine in a changing health service, in Gabe, J., Calnan, M. and Bury, M. *The Sociology of the Health Service*, Routledge, London.

Evans, S., Ewing, K. and Nolan, P. (1992) Industrial relations and the

British Economy in the 1990s; Mrs Thatcher's Legacy, *Journal of Management Studies*, **29**, Sept. 1992, 571–89.

Fielding, A. (1988) Professional elites and the state in privatising Britain, in Thakuar, R.N. (ed.) *Elites: Paradigm and Change in Transnational Perspective*, Indian Political Institute.

Fox, N.J. (1993) *Postmodernism Sociology and Health*, Open University Press, Milton Keynes.

Freidson, E. (1986) *Professional Powers*, Chicago University Press, Chicago.

Gabe, J., Calnan, N. and Bury, M. (1991) *The Sociology of the Health Service*, Routledge, London.

Gabriel, Y. (1988) *Working Lives in Catering*, Routledge, Kegan & Paul, London.

Gallie, D., Marsh, C. and Vogler, C. (1994) *Social Change and the Experience of Unemployment*, Oxford University Press, Oxford.

Garrahan, P. (1992) *The Nissan Enigma: Flexibility at Work in a Local Economy*, Mansell, London.

General Household Survey, as Quoted in Social Trends (1991), HMSO, London.

Gershuny, J. (1983) *The New Service Economy*, Frances Pinter, London.

Gittens, D. (1982) *Fair Sex*, Hutchinson, London.

Goffman, E. (1961) *Asylums: Essays on the social situation of Mental Patients and other inmates*, Doubleday & Co, New York.

Goldthorpe, J., Lockwood, D., Bechhofer, F. and Platt, J. (1968) *The Affluent Worker: Industrial Attitudes and Behaviour*, Cambridge University Press, Cambridge.

Goldthorpe, J. *et al.* (1987) *Social Mobility and Class Structure in Modern Britain*, Oxford University Press, Oxford.

Halmos, P. (1970) *The Personal Service Society*, Constable, London.

Handy, C. (1984) *The Future of Work: A Guide to a Changing Society*, Blackwell, Oxford.

Herzberg, F., Mausner, B. and Snyderman, B. (1959) *The Motivation to Work*, Wiley, New York.

Illich, I. (1975) *Medical Nemesis: The Expropriation of Health*, Calder & Boyers, London.

Jahoda, M. (1982) *Employment and Unemployment: A Social and Psychological Analysis*, Cambridge University Press, Cambridge.

Jacobson, B., Smith, A. and Whitehead, M. (1991) *The Nation's Health: A Strategy for the Nineties*, King Edward's Hospital Fund, London.

Knox, S.S., Theorell, T., Svensonn, J.C. and Waller, D. (1985) The relation of social support and working environment to medical variables associated with elevated blood pressure in young males: a structural model. *Social Science and Medicine*, **21**, 525–31.

Kumar, K. (1978) *Prophecy and Progress*, Allen Lane, London.

Likert, R. (1961) *New Patterns of Management*, McGraw Hill, New York.

McGregor, D. (1960) *The Human Side of Enterprise*, McGraw Hill, New York.

Maslow, A. (1957) *Motivation and Personality*, Harper & Row, New York.

Marx, K. (1844) Economic and philosophical manuscripts, in McLellan, D. (1977) (ed.) *Karl Marx: Selected Writings*, Oxford University Press, Oxford.

Mills, A.J. and Murgatroyd, S.J. (1991) *Organisational Rules*, Open University Press, Milton Keynes.

Morgan, G. (1986) *Images of Organisation*, Sage, London.

Morgan, M. (1991) The doctor-patient relationship, in Scambler, G. (ed.) *Sociology as Applied to Medicine*, Bailliere Tindall, London.

Pilgrim, D. and Rogers, A. (1993) *A Sociology of Mental Health and Illness*, Open University Press, Milton Keynes.

Portwood, D. (1985) The quiescence of the unemployed: a sociological perspective, *Journal of Community Studies*.

Reed, M.I. (1992) *The Sociology of Organisations: Themes, Perspectives and Prospects*, Harvester, London.

Roethlisberger, F. J. and Dickson, W. J. (1939), *Management and the Worker*, Harvard University Press, Cambridge, MA.

Rose, M. (1975) *Industrial Behaviour: Theoretical Developments since Taylor*, Allen Lane, Harmondsworth.

Silverman, D. (1970) *The Theory of Organisation*, Heinemann, London.

Social Trends (1993) (ed.) J. Church, HMSO, London.

Storey, J. (1992) Human resource management in the public sector, in Salaman, G. (ed.) *Human Resource Strategies*, Sage, London.

Taylor, F.W. (1911) *The Principles of Scientific Management*, Harper & Row, New York.

Thompson, P. (1989) *The Nature of Work*, Macmillan, Basingstoke.

Watson, T.J. (1987) *Sociology, Work and Industry*, Routledge & Kegan Paul, London.

Weber, M. (1968) *Economy and Society*, Bedminster, New York.

Weber, M. (1991) *The Protestant Ethic and the Spirit of Capitalism*, Harper Collins Academic, London.

Whitehead, M. (1987) *The Health Divide*, Health Education Authority, London.

Willmott, P. and Young, M. (1973) *The Symmetrical Family*, Routledge & Kegan Paul, London.

5

The quality of working life: occupational stress, job-satisfaction and well-being at work

Peter Spurgeon and Fred Barwell

THE SCOPE OF THE CHAPTER

The quality of working life is a topic that has been discussed in many different guises by a range of experts from a variety of disciplines. Those with an interest in management theory, sociology, industrial relations and organizational behaviour have often debated the ways in which our working lives are structured and the influences upon us at the organizational and societal levels.

Recent changes in the fundamental structure and distribution of work have increasingly focused attention on the central issue of what work means to people. As unemployment continues to rise in the UK, more people are learning first-hand that work is central not only in meeting survival needs but also in meeting people's personal needs for affiliation, self-development and belonging. However, these needs are not always automatically met either in or out of employment and if their expression is thwarted then there are often negative consequences.

In modern industrial society work plays a major role in the lives of most of its members, most obviously providing financial reward that influences the quality of lifestyle. Work also conveys a sense of personal status and identity and for many offers important opportunities for self-development and enhancing self-esteem. The many pressures experienced by the unemployed, sadly reflected in increased suicide rates, is testimony to the potentially devastating impact of the loss of a work role. However, those in work are also subject to pressures. These include individual pressures to perform as well as cultural pressures to attain success in more competitive, more efficient and leaner organizations. These multiple demands at work can leave many individuals suffering from stress and there is a growing concern with the increasing rates of stress-related illnesses. From the 1960s and onwards to the present day, there has been a growing recognition of the importance of identifying stress at work, understanding its causes and consequences and examining strategies to minimize its impact.

This chapter focuses on well-being at work and adopts a broad view of physical and psychological health. A wide perspective is important since it can be misleading not to encompass both clinical states (i.e., neurotic and psychotic psychiatric conditions) and non-clinical states (i.e., impaired job satisfaction and poor self-esteem) in examining health at work.

One significant change over the last 20 years is the increasing recognition of the role that psychosocial factors play in the development and maintenance of physical illness. As Harvey (1988) has observed, it is simply not enough to understand the mechanical processes of disease and illness. In addition, it is essential to understand the social and psychological context that guides individual behaviour, since it is these factors that make some people more prone to illness than others. These days, psychology and medicine are increasingly coupled in assessing individual well-being. This chapter discusses the physical and psychological consequences of work but places more emphasis on the psychological (rather than the medical or sociological) perspective. Consequently, the focus of the chapter is predominantly on the individual employee, his or her personal stressors and his or her attitudinal and behavioural reactions.

MENTAL HEALTH AND WELL-BEING AT WORK

As Warr and Wall (1975) have observed, societies should be measured in terms of their psychological as well as their material success. However, it is far more difficult to measure psychological success than it is to measure concrete wealth. The idea that sources of work stress can sometimes produce job dissatisfaction, mental ill health, heart disease, accident occurrence, alcohol abuse and social and emotional problems is being increasingly supported in a wide range of research findings.

Because health is as much a mental as a physical state it has proved difficult to define. Although the orthodox medical approach is to define health as the absence of disease or symptoms, many believe that this definition is too physically biased and prefer to view health as a positive state of well-being of both the body and the mind (Beric Wright, 1991). Despite this holistic emphasis on psychological as well as physical factors in defining health, the issue of defining and understanding 'mental health' remains difficult and confusing. Typically, those who have attempted to erect definitions (Jahoda, 1958; Kornhauser, 1965) propose a mixture of factual and value statements which attempt to capture the key features of 'mental health', although no definitions are completely satisfactory.

All too often lay people associate mental ill health only with extreme forms of psychological disturbance, but in reality mental ill health may present itself in many common ways. Specific psychological or emotional problems can include everyday issues such as alcohol and drug abuse, anxiety and depression, loneliness and compulsive behaviours. Whatever form these problems take, for the individual sufferer it means that their happiness and effectiveness both socially and at work is always impaired.

Sometimes the 'mental health' issue is tackled by examining an individual's 'adjustment' to their social and occupational environment. However, some psychologists think that these 'adjustment' criteria tend to have an uncomfortable overlap with notions of conformity. Since many neurotics can suffer a great deal from constricted overconforming, the use of adjustment criteria to define 'mental health' may carry negative connotations. To complicate matters further, it is clear that cultural (and sub-cultural or organizational) norms may themselves be psychologically unhealthy and consequently represent an inappropriate metric for defining 'normal' mental health.

A more confident approach to defining 'normality' is the identification of positive characteristics associated with 'mental health'. Although attempts to erect universal standards of mental health do not clearly differentiate between the normal and the abnormal, they are useful in so far as they highlight those traits that normal people tend to possess to a greater degree than abnormal people. For example, most psychologists would agree that the mentally healthy individual has a realistic perception of reality, is self-aware, can voluntarily control his or her behaviour, is socially effective, has adequate self-esteem, is able to form affectionate relationships and is actively productive. Different 'schools' emphasize the importance of different aspects of mental health and consequently focus on different methods to achieve a variety of 'mental health' objectives.

Whatever stance is adopted, clearly psychological well-being at work is important for several enduring reasons. First, since the vast majority of people will always have to work for their living, work may be seen as a desirable end in itself. Second, it is clear that work is of central importance to people and is organized in many ways to satisfy people's requirements for companionship, achievement and gain. In addition to these worker-oriented reasons for pursuing well-being at work, there are those arguments concerned with the development of more effective organizations. In simple terms, people who feel more positively toward their work are more effective at undertaking what is required of them. Those who are stressed, alienated or bored to distraction are generally believed not to be happy or effective employees and these eroding effects can occur across all types and level of occupation.

THE EXTENT OF THE PROBLEM

Illnesses such as mental health, coronary heart disease, strokes and cancers are acknowledged killers in the Western world. These have been increasing over the last 30 years in most industrialized nations (Kasl and Cooper, 1987) and, alongside this, the recognition that the workplace can be extremely stressful has implicated stress as a causal factor in maintaining unhealthy lifestyles and consequent manifestation of illness and disease (Elliott and Eisdorfer, 1982). Furthermore, there has been a shift in some attitudes towards psychological ill health. As people became better educated and more informed, so it was seen that psychosomatic illness and poor mental health were not bizarre and isolated phenomena but conditions that may well affect a very large proportion of the population at some point in their life. Finally, there is a growing understanding that health does not just mean the absence of disease or infirmity but is also a state of physical, mental and social well-being (WHO, 1986). All these issues combined to stimulate interest and research to understand more about the processes involved in stress.

In the course of a year one in ten of the population of the UK (at least six million people) will suffer from some form of mental illness and most of those who are affected are in the working population. It is difficult to obtain precise figures for the incidence of mental disease although MIND has estimated that a quarter of GP consultations at any one time are related to some form of mental distress.

The cost of absence from work because of psychological and emotional problems is enormous and the burden placed on business and industry is immense. Compensation claims for job-related stress have been steadily increasing, and in the United States account for about 14%–15% of all occupational disease claims in 1989 (compared with under 5% in 1979).

Time off work due to stress-related illnesses is estimated to have increased by 500% since the mid–1950s (Beric Wright, 1991). In 1989 in the UK (the last year for which data is available) the total cost of mental illness (including the cost to the NHS) was approaching £7 billion and 80 million working days were lost due to sickness absence certified as mental illness (Waldgrave, 1992).

It has become clear that organizations cannot compete successfully when they are faced with negative behaviours within their workforce. Sutherland (1990) lists several problems that may motivate organizations to tackle sources of stress:

- high turnover
- absenteeism
- poor employee relations
- high accident rates
- decreased performance
- low morale
- increasing litigation

All these problems may be said to be linked to job-related stress.

McLean (1980) has stated that medical practitioners believe that 50%–70% of all illnesses are partly caused through stress. Tension, job dissatisfaction and withdrawal behaviours (i.e., absenteeism, turnover intentions and actual turnover) have repeatedly been demonstrated as correlates of role conflict and role ambiguity (Breaugh, 1981). Each of these problems can be directly linked to role stress. Miner and Brewer (1976) have found poor mental health is a major cause of absenteeism, while Steers and Rhodes (1978) have gone as far as to suggest that absenteeism is healthy for the organization as it allows the employee a break from the stressful work situation.

There is overwhelming evidence that both individuals and organizations need to take the problems of ill health at work very seriously indeed.

THE CENTRAL ROLE OF THE SELF-CONCEPT

Our emotional state influences the ways in which we view ourselves and our relationships with others. One influential attempt to understand human personality is rooted in what has been called the theory of the 'self-concept'. Clearly, the sense of self is a subjective experience and psychoanalysts have recognized that the sense of 'me' develops from an individual's pattern of psychological growth, and in particular their evaluations of their interactions with others.

One recurring theme in many definitions of mental health is the notion that good mental health demands that workers plot a middle course between two consequences. On the one hand, if they want too much compared to what they can achieve the result will be defeat and frustration. On the other hand, if they want too little then their existence will become drab, colourless and low in self-esteem.

William James was the first psychologist to tackle seriously the issues of establishing the importance of the self-concept as something that could be studied objectively. In his monumental work of 1890, *The Principles of Psychology,* James described the factors that determine any individual's self-regard or self-esteem. In evaluating themselves, a person's feelings of self-worth depend to a large extent on how they appraise themselves in relation to others who are in the 'same boat'. James argued that self-esteem all depends on what you see yourself as, and he calls these appraisals 'pretensions'.

An Olympic athlete who 'only' wins a silver medal may see himself as a complete failure because he did not achieve the gold medal. His self-esteem may be severely shaken because he has set his personal goal to be a gold medallist. Using James' formula, self-esteem = success / pretensions, it is apparent that this athlete's loss of self-esteem would have been the exact opposite had he not defined success so highly. Had he defined success as achieving a bronze medal, the identical performance would have resulted in enhancing his self-regard. The point that James is making is that expectations are self-imposed and refer to an individual's personal level of goal-setting and aspirations.

However, for many people the appropriate opportunities for fully developing positive subjective feelings of uniqueness are not always available. This potential for effective personal growth can be curtailed or stunted by unfavourable circumstances in the home and work environment. In restrictive or deprived work conditions, negative emotional responses such as anger, aggression and hostility are only to be expected and they are a natural and healthy reaction to oppressive work. However, negative feelings often do not conveniently confine themselves to the situations that have created these conditions of psychological poverty, but can become the predominant psychological feature in the individual's whole life pattern.

Events and transactions that lower self-esteem or produce a sense of loneliness or hopelessness are those that tend to predispose individuals to have a lowered resistance to illness and to reduce their effectiveness at work.

PERSONAL VALUES, CAREER CHOICE AND ADJUSTMENT

The ways in which people select and progress through their careers reflects and reinforces individual adjustment to work and is consequently an important factor in determining mental health. In these times of economic recession, the issue of choosing suitable work is for many far less pressing than finding any work at all. Unfortunately, for increasing numbers of people occupational choice is not a practical reality. Where occupational choice remains a real possibility, the decision-making process has often been portrayed as an expression of the individual's value-structure and personality rather than being a rationally based evaluation of available alternatives.

The persistent belief that occupational choice reflects and reinforces personality has led to the corollary that those indi-

viduals in the same sorts of job share common needs and values
and also tend to have similar sorts of personalities. For example,
in a series of studies Reich and Geller (1976a and 1976b) have
provided evidence that different occupations are associated with
different personality characteristics. For two caring occupations,
nursing and social work, these researchers found different patterns of self-descriptions in completing the Adjective Check List
(Gough and Heillbron, 1965). Nurses described themselves in a
way that suggested that their choice of nursing as a career is in
part the outcome of strongly denied dependency needs. In contrast, social workers tended to portray themselves in ways that
suggested that the desire to do well is a stronger motivator in
their career choice than the desire to be nurturant and care for
others.

Super (Super *et al.*, 1963) is the dominant theorist who identified the self-concept as critical in shaping an individual's choice
of job. Super sees vocational development as developing a 'self-
concept' as a worker and considers that the process of establishing a career occurs in three broad stages:

- Formation or growth stage (birth–14) when development takes
  place through identification with key figures in family and in
  school and during which choice is initially dominated (up to
  the age of 10 by needs and fantasies. These fantasies increasingly give way to career choices guided by likes, interests,
  perceived abilities and job requirements.
- Translation or exploration stage (age 15–24) when the self-
  concept begins to be translated into occupational terms and
  role try-outs and occupational exploration takes place until a
  seemingly appropriate field is selected and a trial 'job-for-life'
  period occurs.
- Implementation or establishment stage (age 25–44) when effort
  is made to establish and stabilize the career role. There may
  be one or two changes until life work is found or it becomes
  clear that the life work will be a succession of jobs.

The development of the self-concept takes place through life's
experiences and is moulded by the reactions of others. Super
suggests that satisfaction in an occupation depends upon the
extent to which the occupation enables the individual to play
the sort of role he or she wants to play.

After achieving a stable work role, Herzberg (1966) has argued that mental health at work requires two further sorts of psychological development. First, the individual must adjust to the demands of the work environment to minimize the impact of negative states. Second, an individual must achieve psychological growth at work and this may occur through some of the following five overlapping processes. If undertaken in an authentic fashion, all five approaches can increase the individual's 'psychological tissue'.

1. Increasing the acquisition of work-related knowledge;
2. Structuring what is learnt at work through organizing and integrating experiences;
3. Producing original thoughts or things through personal creativity;
4. Dealing with uncertainty and real-world complexity;
5. Developing an individuality that is not overdetermined by group dependence and conformity.

Clearly the current work environment is highly influential in shaping attitudes and behaviours at work, although apparently pre-employment experiences are also powerful influences on how the workplace is perceived and reacted to. Early family experiences (particularly impaired parent-child relationships) can later affect job attitudes and relationships with superiors (Thomas and Duszynski, 1974; Firth, 1985). Physical and emotional deprivation in childhood, poor parental models and low self-esteem can all act as early agents that make people more vulnerable to work adjustment in later life.

These early predisposing factors may heighten the probability that later circumstances can act to precipitate the onset of mental illness. As well as maladaptive psychological disturbances, physical and social factors as divergent as malignant diseases, injuries, separation, divorce, threat of unemployment or redundancy, can all precipitate individuals into mental illness.

It is clear that the psychological and emotional problems that may find expression in the workplace usually have multiple causes. Generally, the causes of psychological illness can ultimately be traced back to psychological, social or genetic factors. For example, the very severe psychotic illnesses such as psychotic depression and schizophrenia have a strong genetic contribution whereas this is not so for the non-psychotic illnesses such as depression or anxiety which are more likely to occur as a reaction to mental or physical stress (including physical illness). The working environment itself can act in a stressful or supporting way and the potential stressful impact of work on individuals' well-being will be examined in more detail later in this chapter.

JOB SATISFACTION

Although perceptions of the workplace clearly influence feelings of well-being and attitudes to the job and these factors have been frequently explored, the concept of job satisfaction is only poorly understood. Contrary to popular expectation, most studies seem to find that people are relatively satisfied with their jobs. For example, Quinn and Staines (1979) report that within one survey that has been carried out annually for more than 20 years, over 80% of employees appear reasonably happy with their jobs and life at work.

However, this comforting view of a satisfied and a contented workforce may be more apparent than real. Lying just beneath the surface of many reported aggregated indicators of job satisfaction there are several reasons why it may not be as widespread as some surveys seem to show. First, it seems that those who dislike their jobs tend to change them and the typical research finding that length of service is associated with job satisfaction supports this view. Second, over the years, people tend to adjust to their working conditions and this increases their tolerance to work conditions. Interestingly, Parlmore (1969) found that job satisfaction was a better predictor of the age at which people would die than a range of more obvious predictors including measures of physical health, smoking habits and economic position and security.

Clearly job satisfaction is a powerful predictive concept that is also practically very important since a large body of evidence suggests that those who have a positive set of attitudes to their work behave differently from those who see work from a negative viewpoint. However, reliably and validly assessing people's reactions to work is not always as easy as it might at first appear. Essentially, this is the case because people tend to keep their attitudes to themselves and are naturally reluctant to let their managers become aware of their honest opinions since this may jeopardize their relationships at work or even the security of their job. To overcome this natural reluctance to be honest, assessment of employee reactions often takes place either indirectly through examining behaviourial indices such as absenteeism or turnover or through self-report in surveys or questionnaires.

SOME CAUSES OF JOB SATISFACTION

Although aggregated job-satisfaction data is often interpreted to support the idea that people are generally well-satisfied at work, there is a great deal of difference between individuals with respect to their levels of job satisfaction. This means that morale and motivation are very high in some quarters and virtually absent in others. These differences can occur between organizations or even between different departments in the same organization.

Understanding job satisfaction is a complex undertaking and despite a great deal of investigation the causes and consequences of negative attitudes to the workplace are far from fully understood. In simple terms, job satisfaction or job dissatisfaction depends in part on two sorts of factor: factors to do with the workplace and factors to do with the individual. Working conditions that provide challenging (but not overwhelming) tasks and reward systems (i.e. pay, bonuses and promotions) that are perceived as not only fair but also under employee control tend to result in high job satisfaction. Similarly, high job satisfaction generally goes hand-in-hand with a comfortable working environment. Uncomfortable work environments are high in physical and psychological stress and often lead to job dissatisfaction.

Besides these external causes of job satisfaction, there are other internal causes related to the personality or disposition of the individual employee. Individuals with a positive self-image, those who are able to withstand stress and those who are high in status or seniority, tend to report higher levels of job satisfaction than those who have low self-esteem, low tolerance and low status. The patterns of causality related to these findings are not always clear but it seems fair to say that those individuals who are happy and well-adjusted off the job also tend to be satisfied on the job as well.

Often it is difficult to predict the effects of high and low job satisfaction on work behaviour and this difficulty stems in part from the fact that job satisfaction is not a single phenomena but rather represents a cluster of related attitudes. Of course, attitudes do not always affect behaviour in a clear-cut way and this may account for the fact that only modest relationships are typically found between job satisfaction and such factors as absenteeism and turnover. Similarly, despite frequent attempts to demonstrate that satisfaction and performance or productivity are positively related, there is little or no evidence to suggest that there is such a link. This implies that programmes designed to increase satisfaction at work cannot be expected to have an extensive affect on job performance.

One common source of psychological stress at work centres on the interpersonal relations between co-workers and supervisors. Friendly, positive relations tend to produce high satisfaction, as does the opportunity to participate in work-related decisions. These interpersonal factors are discussed in greater detail later in the chapter.

THE NATURE OF STRESS

Like job satisfaction, stress is not a precise term and it is used in slightly different ways by different authors. This means that confusion surrounds both its meaning and attempts to measure it. Approaches to the study of stress have taken different forms, as shown below:

- as an organism's response to a demand or to events that challenge it (Seyle, 1976);
- as an event external to the individual that places demands upon him/her (Kahn, 1964);
- as a characteristic of the environment that poses a threat to the individual (Caplan *et al.*, 1975);
- as a state that results from a misfit between a person's skills and the demands placed upon him/her (McGrath, 1976).

Stress is seen either as something external to the individual, or as an internal state or as an interaction between the two.

Early attempts to examine stress concentrated on the physiological aspects of the stress response, although in time psychological components were increasingly incorporated in stress models. However, the wide range and variability of the reactions of different people to apparently similar situations have constrained the development of a simple universally acceptable

model of stress. Cox (1978) added a useful insight in sugg
that 'stress has to be perceived or recognised by man'. Fro
stance has emerged the consensus view that understanding ьисss
requires that an interpretative element is introduced into the
process by which different individuals respond to their
environment.

Newton (1989) saw this interpretation as the subjective
appraisal of the demands made on the individual and argued
that it is a vital aspect in understanding stress. From this perspective, it becomes easier to understand why people react differently
in certain settings. An interesting corollary of making subjective-
event appraisal a key feature of a stress model is that it becomes
apparent that stress is not always negative and can provide a
positive or constructive influence. Life without stimulation or
challenge would be intolerably boring and reasonable amounts
of pressure heighten our arousal and performance. It is only
when an individual feels that the amount of pressure being
applied is excessive that the outcome becomes potentially damaging (BMA, 1992).

This notion of positive enhancement is described by Quick
and Quick (1984) as a process by which individuals attempt to
maintain a balance in ongoing variations in stress levels. This
occurs not only when the demand on a person exceeds capability
or the desired level, but also when capability exceeds demand;
in other words when boredom arises. Clearly, the individual is
not a passive component in the stress process since he or she
can conceptualize surrounding events and situations in many
different ways.

From this perspective of the individual as an active component
in the stress situation, several approaches arise by which the
individual may attempt to manage stressful environments. A key
factor in the negative impact of stress is the perceived control, or
more accurately the lack of perceived control, over the provoking
situation (Landsbergis, 1988). Similarly, individual strategies
such as defence mechanisms, aimed at improving the 'fit' of the
individual to the environment, are active attempts to restructure
the stress environment.

However, the person-environment fit approach to understanding stress is not without its critics. Handy (1988) and Hobfall
(1989) both suggest that the emphasis on the perception or
appraisal process merely leads to a view that everyone is differ-

ent and shifts the emphasis of research to defining individual personality characteristics that allow some people to thrive while others suffer. They are also concerned that an overemphasis on appraisal mechanisms has the potential danger of detracting attention from the proper consideration of the sources of stress within organizations. These stressors may be conveniently ignored since experience of them is always mediated by the individual.

The experience of stress

We have seen that it is possible for the individual to act upon the person-environment fit and, if successful, adjust the situation appropriately. However, this may not succeed and the individual may then become subject to longer term strains and may start to demonstrate the symptoms of stress. There is a danger in simply listing sets of symptoms partly because individual reactions are so different and partly because it might suggest that specific symptoms have a specific one-to-one relationship with a source of stress.

Nonetheless there are some crude classifications that are useful. The first category is really a short-term response to stress: 'the fight or flight response' is well-understood physiologically. The release of adrenalin and steroids associated with stress causes various physiological changes, such as:

- increased blood pressure;
- increased muscle tension;
- increased sweating;
- release of glucose and fats into the blood;
- dry mouth.

These physiological changes can be directly related to the observed outcomes of stress in individuals.

The second category traverses both short and long-term responses, being primarily psychological: here we find such symptoms as anxiety, depression and job dissatisfaction. A final level is behaviourial where performance is adversely affected in some way; for example, behaviourial problems can be manifested as absenteeism from work or difficulties within personal life.

Despite the earlier comments in this chapter about the impact of stress on individual health, there is less clear-cut evidence about the links between the affects of stress and long illness. However, studies have suggested an association stress and the following illnesses:

- long-term depression;
- ulcers;
- allergies;
- headaches;
- coronary heart disease;
- cancer;
- asthma.

While there is controversy about the precise causal link between stress and particular illnesses, it may be useful to look briefly at two conditions where stress is acknowledged as a primary cause; 'burn-out' and post-traumatic stress disorder (PTSD). Although individuals may adopt superficially successful methods of coping with stress, it might be that the very act of coping exacts a toll upon the person so as to impair professional functioning.

The term 'burn-out' was first used by Freudenberger (1984) to describe a syndrome especially common among health workers. The syndrome, although lacking a precise definition, is usually seen as having three components:

- emotional exhaustion (tiredness, irritability, depression);
- depersonalization (poor relationships with others);
- low productivity (with accompanying feelings of low achievement).

The initial link with health workers is interesting and will be discussed more generally later in this chapter.

Post-traumatic stress disorder is a specific anxiety disorder that occurs following a stressful or traumatic event. The key component seems a re-experiencing of the traumatic event at a later date. The syndrome is particularly associated with direct experience of major disasters but it can occur with apparently less significant everyday events. In the long term, sufferers tend to manifest social and occupational dysfunctioning as well as psychiatric illness. It is again of special interest to the medical world because of their exposure to the victims of disasters.

SOME SOURCES OF STRESS AT WORK

Individuals have quite different orientations to work and attribute value on varying components of their overall lifework pattern. Therefore it is possible for individuals to perceive the same job in quite different ways. People bring personality traits, coping strategies and interpersonal factors into the workplace and each of these can have a moderating effect on the source of stress (the stressor) within the job. The impact of these various moderators will be reviewed in the next section.

Differences between individuals' reactions to different aspects of the working environment make the classification of stressor types difficult. Nevertheless, it is possible to identify potential sources of stress within the workplace. Sutherland and Cooper (1988) provide an excellent overview of these stressors, categorizing them into five major types:

1. Factors intrinsic to the job:
   - poor physical working conditions (due to noise, vibration, temperature, ventilation, humidity, lighting, hygiene and climate);
   - work overload and underload (qualitative and quantitative);
   - time pressures;
   - responsibility for lives.
2. Role of the individual in the organization:
   - role ambiguity/conflict;
   - image of occupational role;
   - boundary conflicts.
3. Career development:
   - overpromotion;
   - underpromotion;
   - lack of job security;
   - thwarted ambition.
4. Relationships at work:
   - poor relations with boss, subordinates or colleagues;
   - difficulties in delegating responsibility.
5. Organizational structure and climate:
   - little or no participation in decision-making;
   - restrictions on behaviour (budgets etc.);
   - office politics;
   - lack of effective consultation.

It is not possible to provide in-depth coverage of all these within this chapter but selective examples of each suggests the sort of stress process involved.

Factors intrinsic to the job

The first component of this category is concerned with the physical demands of the workplace. Kornhauser (1965) reported that poor mental well-being was directly related to unpleasant work conditions, the necessity to work fast, expenditure of physical effort and inconvenient hours. Typical of work in this area is the concern expressed towards unwanted noise in the workplace. Although noise can be quantified and objectively assessed, there is a strong view that reaction to noise remains a subjective phenomenon. Noise, though, is typically associated with fatigue, headaches, irritability and inability to concentrate, increased sound isolation, open hostility and overt aggression (James, 1983). It is interesting how high domestic noise irritates many people (e.g. barking dogs, loud radios, etc.). However, within the work context there is a clear interaction between the task and the source of noise, thus making it difficult to disentangle sources of stress or noise alone or noise in conjunction with task demands and other poor working conditions.

Other stressors within this physical-environment category include vibration, lighting and extremes of temperature. Unpleasant working conditions, due to heat, cold, noise and vibration were a significant predictor of job dissatisfaction among many workers in the UK and Dutch sectors of the North Sea (Sutherland and Cooper, 1986).

The second component of this first category, that of task demands, has also provided a major impetus to stress research. Shiftwork and nightwork are a key issue here, with some 20% of the working population estimated to be working a shift system not by choice but of necessity (Cooper and Smith, 1986). Generalization is difficult, but reports of fatigue and gastrointestinal troubles appear higher in the shiftwork population (Rutenfranz *et al.*, 1974). There are an enormous number of variations of shiftwork arrangements (Singer, 1985 reports some 487 different patterns) and this source of variability, coupled with disparate individual reactions to shiftwork (both physiological and psychological), makes it difficult in practice to recommend ideal shift patterns.

The final major category within job demands is represented by the complex concept of workload. Both physical and mental overload – that is, simply having too much to do – is a potent source of stress at work. Time pressures and deadlines emphasize the impact of load. Quantitative overload is significantly related to absenteeism and escapist drinking (Margolis, Kroes and Quinn, 1974). Although of slightly lower intensity, there is a similar degree of stress associated with quantitative underload. In particular, boredom produces a lack of attention that results in errors and potential exposure to hazards. There is also a parallel process involving qualitative overload and workload where the demands of the task simply do not fit the capacity of the employee. Both overload and underload result in a lowering of self-esteem.

The role of the individual in the organization

Miles and Perrault (1976) have discussed classifications of role tensions in some detail, although the two most often cited are role conflict and role ambiguity. The individual with role conflict is stressed by trying to meet the competing demands of other members of the organization or indeed conflicts with his or her personal values. Role ambiguity is more concerned with situations where an employee is unclear about what is required in the role or does not properly understand the expectations of how he or she is expected to perform. It is probably true to say that this type of stressor affects higher level, more complex jobs although this is not exclusively the case.

Relationships and interpersonal demands

Poor relationships at work can be characterized as having low trust, low levels of supportiveness and low interest in problem-solving within the organization. In this sense, negative relationships at work are parallel to many aspects of interpersonal conflict in life. Poor relationships within a group of co-workers are a common source of stress, but perhaps of more immediate impact is a poor interpersonal relationship between an individual and his or her superior. Over-supervision, rigid monitoring and a concern only with task performance can contribute to feelings of job pressure. Cooper and Marshall (1978) suggest that for some technically oriented supervisors a concern with interpersonal aspects of work relationships may be seen as rather trivial and perhaps indicative of weakness.

Quick and Quick (1984) identify five specific forms of interpersonal stressors:

1. Status incongruence: where incongruence between the status of a job as perceived by an employee and what that same employee believes it should be may lead to frustration;
2. Social density: where inadequate workspace due to overcrowding or isolation affects performance, satisfaction and morale;
3. Abrasive personalities: who may unwittingly cause stress to others because they ignore feelings and sensitivities in their interactions with others. This is difficult on a peer basis but is even more threatening when a boss or superior is involved.
4. Leadership style: this could be linked to personal qualities but more generally is concerned with the lack of feedback, lack of support and failure to offer routes for participation;
5. Group pressure: this is a very powerful phenomenon and well-documented (e.g. Smith, Colligan and Tasto, 1982). It can cause great individual distress where the pressure of the group conflicts with the values and beliefs of one of its members.

Career development

This potential stressor applies to certain types of jobs more than others. Although the term 'career' is not really applicable to many blue collar occupations, there are some aspects of this stressor that may apply to many people, especially in the current economic climate. Sadly, fear of job loss and redundancy are increasingly common features of working life and can be a potent source of serious health problems (e.g., ulcers, colitis: Cobb and Kasl, 1977; and emotional distress: Smith *et al.*, 1981).

Somewhat less dramatic but still a potential source of stress is the issue of promotion. Some individuals may be placed in situations well beyond their capabilities while others suffer the frustration, low self-esteem and depression of being unable to advance.

Organizational structure and climate

This possible stressor is principally concerned with how the organization treats its employees. A central factor is the level of involvement and participation offered, with a lack of autonomy and control over one's own work associated with increased risks of coronary heart disease (Karasek, 1979).

INDIVIDUAL MODERATORS OF STRESS

The factors discussed in the previous section may be present within an organization to varying degrees, but the way in which individuals perceive these situations will be modified by a variety of individual and social factors. The current opinion is that environments are not inherently stressful although it is probably self-evident that some situations will be perceived as more adverse by most people and therefore might be classified as potentially very stressful. Nevertheless, there has been considerable research effort directed to finding why some people react to stressors in markedly different forms.

The obvious concern with stress generally is, of course, based largely on the predicted link to poor health. However, even this relationship is subject to potential moderation by other factors. For example, Paffenbarger, Wolf and Notkin (1966) reported that personality scores on levels of anxiety and neuroticism for a group of students were predictive of future fatal coronary heart disease. More generally, other personality characteristics identified as modifiers of response to stress include introversion-extroversion (Brief *et al.*, 1981), anxiety (Chan, 1977) and tolerance for ambiguity (Ivancevich and Matteson, 1980).

Perhaps the most significant of the personality-based modifiers is the evidence accumulated about the Type A and Type B personality and its link to vulnerability to stress. The area was defined in the 1950s by Friedman and Rosenman (1959) who noted a distinct behaviourial pattern within their coronary heart disease patients. The typical Type A personality is described as work-oriented, high achievers who are very competitive and impatient. Of course, this is a pattern of behaviour that many organizations might value and indeed such individuals are often very successful. Also, it may be that Type A individuals also seek out stressful work environments that meet their personal needs for challenge and achievement. Nonetheless, there is a general view that there is a difference between Type A and Type B individuals with Type As being more disposed to suffer negative stress outcomes. Of course, if this were consistently the case, we could identify Type A personalities and conclude that they have an enhanced risk of stress-related illness. However, recent evidence suggests that the Type A/Type B distinction is not quite as clear-cut as it once seemed. There appears to be a strong link between social class and whether an individual is Type A or B, while Haynes, Feinlieb and Eaker (1981) only found a link with coronary heart disease with white collar groups. Johnston, Cook and Shaper (1987) in a six-year study failed to find any distinction in levels of heart disease between the two groups.

Another stress moderator is the 'locus of control' construct. This is essentially concerned with the degree of control that individuals perceive they exercise over events. Those with an internal orientation are motivated by their own actions and believe life events are under their control, while those with an external orientation believe that others influence events and consequently have a greater tendency to feel helpless. Clearly it is a natural dimension to see it as a moderator of stress. In general, individual orientation provides a much greater chance of dealing with stressors (Blaney, 1985; Payne, 1988), whilst Perrewe and Ganster (1989) argue that control is important to various positive health outcomes.

Finally, there is evidence that some very specific individual characteristics may interact with experience of stress. Research evidence suggests that women suffer psychological and physiological stressors in the work environment on a rather greater scale than their male counterparts (Hall and Hall, 1980). However, a recent review of the stress literature by Mavtocchio and O'Leary (1989) has fuelled renewed debate in the area since they were unable to detect any gender-based differences in susceptibility to stress. Osipow, Doty and Spokame (1985) found that older employees reported less stress than younger employees and used more coping strategies to deal with stressors.

All these factors contribute to the complexity of determining the outcome of potential stressors on the individual. The evidence presented so far in this chapter has related generally to all types of employee and occupational groups. However, there is nsiderable interest in stress within the medical and caring professions and it is to these we now turn.

STRESS IN THE CARING OCCUPATIONS

As the reforms in the NHS have unfolded, various groups within the health professions have found their existing levels of patient-based stress exacerbated by new pressures of reduced resources, limited staff and raised performance targets. Sutherland and Cooper (1992) specifically examined the sources of stress in General Practitioners following the introduction of a new financial and performance contract. They report some basic causes of stress in GPs as:

- excessive demands and expectations of patients;
- conflict with needs of family and social life;
- discord with partners;
- uncertainty of relationships in the team;
- uncertainty over doctors' role, especially in relationship to non-clinical work;
- preserving image in the community;
- time.

More generally, Elliott-Binns, Bingham and Peile (1992) have explored the impact of stress on the whole primary-care team. They suggest, for example, that nurses within the practice are particularly concerned with role-confusion and their employment position. Interestingly, Hingley, Cooper and Harris (1986) have also examined sources of stress within the nursing profession. Although much has been made of the vocational aspect of choosing nursing as a career (in part to justify low pay levels), it does seem that nurses have a strong commitment to their work tasks and should have well-developed coping strategies. Indeed, the evidence presented by Hingley, Cooper and Harris reinforces this picture. They conclude that:

> Nurses are less likely to feel stress from factors intrinsic to the primary nursing task than by workers relationships, formal structures within the organisation and factors external to their jobs. Indeed, only one area of concern, 'death and dying' is directly related to patient care.

However, a series of further stressors within nursing were identified:

- workload, particularly relating to time pressures, and staff shortages;
- relationships with supervisors, especially the lack of positive feedback;
- home/work conflict, typically a female profession with additional pressures created by working unsocial hours and yet trying to manage a home and family;
- physical resources, relating to unsuitable and inadequate equipment, and a lack of privacy;
- change; this represented a continuing pressure resulting from the major upheavals in the structure and management of the NHS.

The negative feelings of nurses to the increasing financial pressures within the health service can be seen in reported feelings of lack of personal achievement, depression, discouragement and emotional exhaustion with their attempts to continue to provide good patient care under constrained resources (Firth, 1984).

Maslach (1982), recognizing this situation, argues for special training and preparation for working with other people. Evidence of this approach is seen in terms of more counselling skills and bereavement support for nurses. The extent of concern is further reinforced by Burnard (1991) which offers a positive guide to health professionals in dealing with stress. Finally, in considering strategies for dealing with stress it might be appropriate to consider how both organizations and individuals can respond.

INDIVIDUAL AND ORGANIZATIONAL APPROACHES TO COPING WITH STRESS

Throughout this chapter, it has been emphasized that stress is always mediated by the individual's perceptions and that situations that are stressful to some people may be challenging to others. It is generally true, however, that most people view stress as a negative force and can consequently be very defensive about admitting they feel stressed or seeking some form of support. Jenkins (1992) has suggested that we are all a little proud of work pressure or stress but that we are ashamed of this leading to physical or psychological ill health.

Increasingly an individual's capacity to identify the need for and enter appropriate support is a key element in dealing with stress and maintaining a sense of well-being (Dooley, Rook and Catalamo, 1987). Two forms of social-support mechanism have been identified by Carver, Schier and Weintraub (1989). These are:

1. a problem-focused, rational approach that seeks support in the form of guidance, advice, assistance or information;
2. an emotion-focused approach looking for social support in the form of moral support, sympathy and understanding.

The two, although conceptually separate, may of course occur simultaneously. Provision of such support, though, is not always easy even when the need has been identified. First, the support needs to be well directed to the initial issue within the stressor set and evidence suggests that it is likely to be most effective if it is in a form quite familiar to the individual receiving it. There is further evidence, too, that men derive more effective support when it is derived from a work context, while women use external supports to more advantage (Roos and Cohen, 1987).

To some extent the value of social support depends on the level of emotion experienced and the focus of this emotion. Heron (1977) distinguishes four types of emotion commonly expressed during the process of experiencing stress: anger, fear, grief and embarrassment. These reactions may become blurred but the effects of bottling-up these emotions is likely to lead to symptoms such as physical discomfort, muscular pain, poor decision-making, low self-image and setting unattainable targets – thus perpetuating the stress.

There are a range of individually based techniques available such as breathing exercises to control immediate symptoms; meditation exercises to restore the mind and body; and learning to be more assertive in order to counter the negative impact of the stressful environment. Whether a particular approach is used in practice is likely to depend upon availability in a rather haphazard fashion.

The randomness of this *laissez-faire* approach may be lessened by use of a counselling support system. The idea here is that the individual, through the help of the counsellor, can learn to identify stress sources, identify their particular needs and review the appropriateness of support mechanisms. Employers are slowly beginning to recognize the value of the provision of internal counselling services and are locating trained counsellors within their organization. Again, this is an increasing provision with respect to nurses who may experience intense stress through dealing with death and trauma as well as more continuous pressure from job demands.

This type of provision raises the issue of the organizational response to stress. Service managers may be the most difficult to influence towards the value of some form of internal stress-support programme since almost by definition they are likely to have been successful and coped without support. If this attitude pervades the organization, then more junior staff may find difficulties in enrolling on to a programme as it may be taken to indicate failure and therefore the inability to cope with the added pressures inherent within a promotion. This somewhat 'macho' approach also tends to prevent the organization recognizing that its own culture may be part of the problem. This is gradually changing as organizations recognize that people are its key asset and need to be helped to be as effective as possible.

Even when a programme of stress management is offered it needs to be sensitively marketed within the organization. Compulsory attendance is likely to be counter-productive, and if voluntary some non-attenders may be the very people who would most benefit but have not reached the psychological stage of recognizing a need for support (Conrad, 1987).

Organisationally based stress-management programmes are reviewed by Sutherland (1990). She describes the following types:

- Educational/awareness programmes aimed primarily at helping the employee be aware of the links between stress, illness and personal behaviour;
- Assessment-focused programmes that aim to identify individual stress profiles to highlight problem areas, risk environments. This can be done individually or in a group and will review the person's history, work and home context, experiences of stressful events and their coping strategies;
- Skill-building programmes where the focus is more on giving individuals particular skills to help them cope, such as relaxation skills, cognitive restructuring, interpersonal skills such

as assertiveness training, exercise and physical fitness regimes and diet;

- Counselling programmes (as discussed in the previous section);
- Organizational-change approaches that are directed to changing policies and practices within the organization so the individual is subject to less potential stressor because of the cultural shift in the organization.

All the programmes can make a contribution but the style of the introduction into an organization is critical. Nevertheless, tackling occupational stress can be regarded as a worthwhile proposition for both individuals and for organizations (Cooper, 1988). There is real value in intervening in the work situation, especially if the approach is preventive rather than tackling problems when they have become conspicuous. For example, the Control Data Corporation in the USA initiated a 'Staywell' programme for 22,000 employees and their spouses. The programme included programmes to encourage the stopping of smoking, weight control, cardiovascular fitness, stress management and diet improvement. The evaluation demonstrated that those participating in the programmes had significantly reduced healthcare and hospital-stay costs, while those not participating were found twice as likely to be absent from work due to sickness.

In conclusion it is clear that stress is a significant problem for individuals and organizations. Unfortunately, it is a complex problem not susceptible to easy solutions either for the person suffering from stress or for the support agencies attempting to relieve its negative consequences.

REFERENCES

Beric Wright, H. (1991) *Are You Managing Your Health?*, The Industrial Society, London.
Blaney, P.H. (1985) Stress and depression in adults: a critical review, in Field, T.M., McCabe, P.H. and Schmiedeman, N. (eds) *Stress and Coping*, Earlbaum, New Jersey.
BMA (1992) *Stress and the Medical Profession*, Chameleon Press, London.
Breaugh, J.A. (1981) Predicting absenteeism from prior absenteeism and work attitudes. *Journal of Applied Psychology*, **66**(5), 555–60.
Brief, A.P., Sculer, R.S. and Van Self, M.C. (1981) *Managing Job Stress*, Little, Brown, Boston.

Burnard, P. (1991) *Coping with Stress in the Health Professions: A Practical Guide*, Chapman & Hall, London.

Caplan, R.D., Cobb, S., and French, J.R.P. (1975) *Job Demands and Workers Health*, US Government Printing Office, US Department of Health, Education and Welfare, Washington DC.

Carver, C.S., Schier, M.F., and Weintraub, J.K. (1989) Assessing coping strategies: a theoretical based approach. *Journal of Personal and Social Psychology*, **56**(2), 267–83.

Chan, K.B. (1977) Individual differences in reactions to stress and their personality and situational determinants. *Social Science and Medicine*, **11**, 89–103.

Cobb, S. and Kasl, S.V. (1977) *Termination – the consequences of job loss*, HEW Publication, Cincinnati, pp. 77–224.

Conrad, P. (1987) Who comes to work-site wellness programmes? A preliminary review. *Journal of Occupational Medicine*, **29**(4), 317–20.

Cooper, C.L. (1986) Job distress: recent research and the emerging role of the clinical occupational psychologist. *Bulletin of British Psychological Society*, **39**, 325–31.

Cooper, C.L. (1988) Stress in the workplace: recent research evidence, in Pettigrew, A.M. (ed.) *Companies and the Management*, Blackwell, Oxford.

Cooper, C.L. and Marshall, J.C. (1978) *Understanding Executive Stress*, Macmillan, London.

Cooper, C.L. and Smith, M. (1986) *Job Stress and Blue Collar Work*, John Wiley, Chichester.

Cox, T.C. (1978) *Stress*, Macmillan, London.

Dooley, D., Rook, R., and Catalamo, R.C. (1987) Job and non-job stressors and their moderators. *Journal of Occupational Psychology*, **60**, 115–32.

Elliott, G.R. and Eidorfer, C. (eds) (1982) *Stress and Human Health: Analysis and Implications of Research*, Springer, New York.

Elliott-Binns, C., Bingham, L. and Peile, E. (eds) (1992) *Managing Stress in the Primary Care Team*, Blackwell Scientific Publications, Oxford.

Firth, H. (1984) Measures of Staff Support and Adaptation to Work in Long Stay Care. *Annual Progress Report*, Praedhoe Hospital, Northumberland Health Authority.

Firth, J.A. (1985) Personal meanings of occupational stress: cases from the clinic. *Journal of Occupational Psychology*, **58**, 139–42.

Freudenberger, H.J. (1984) Staff burn-out. *Journal of Social Issues*, **30**, 159–65.

Friedman, M. and Rosenman, R.H. (1959) Association of specific overt behaviour patterns with blood and cardio-vascular findings. *Journal of the American Medical Association*, **169**, 1286–96.

Gough, H.G. and Heillbron, A.B. (1965) *Adjective Check List Manual*, Consulting Psychologists Press, Palo Alto.

Hall, D.T. and Hall, F.S. (1980) Stress and the two career couple, in Cooper, C.L. and Payne, R. (eds) *Current Concerns in Occupational Stress*, Wiley, New York.

Handy, J.A. (1988) Theoretical and methodological problems within occupational stress and burnout research. *Human Relations*, **41**(5), 351–69.

Harvey, P. (1988) *Health Psychology*, Longman, Harlow.

Haynes, S.G., Feinlieb, M. and Eaker, E.D. (1981) Type A behaviour and the ten year incidence of coronary heart disease in the Framingham Heart Study, in Rosenman, R.H. (ed.) *Psychosomatic Risk Factors and Coronary Heart Disease: Indication for Specific Preventative Therapy*, Hans Huber, Berne.

Heron, J. (1977) *Catharsis in Human Development*, Human Potential Research Project, University of Surrey, Guildford.

Herzberg, F. (1966) *Work and the Nature of Man*, World Publishing Company, Cleveland, Ohio.

Hingley, P., Cooper, C.L. and Harris, P. (1986) *Stress in Nurse Managers*, King's Fund Centre, London.

Hobfall, S. (1989) *The Ecology of Stress*, Hemisphere, New York.

Ivancevich, J.M. and Matteson, M.T. (1980) *Stress at Work*, Scott Foresman, Glenview, Illinois.

Jahoda, M. (1958) *Current Concepts of Mental Health*, Basic Books, London.

James, D.M. (1983) Noise, in Hockey, R. (ed.) *Stress and Fatigue in Human Performance*, John Wiley, Chichester.

James, W. (1890) *The Principles of Psychology*, Holt, New York.

Jenkins, R. (1992) The prevalence, causes and consequences of mental ill health at work, in Jenkins, R. and Coney, N., *Prevention of Mental Ill Health at Work*, HMSO, London.

Johnston, D.W., Cook, D.G., and Shaper, A.G. (1987) *Type A behaviour and ischaemic heart disease in middle-aged British men*, paper presented at the Society of Behaviourial Medicine, Washington.

Kahn, R.L. (1964) *Role Stress: Studies in Role Conflict and Ambiguity*, John Wiley, New York.

Karasek, R.A. (1979) Job demands, job decision latitude and mental strain: implications for job redesign. *Administrative Science Quarterly*, **24**, 285–306.

Kasl, S. and Cooper, C.L. (1987) *Stress and Health Issues in Research Methodology*, John Wiley, New York.

Kornhauser, A.W. (1965) *Mental Health of the Industrial Worker: A Detroit Study*, Wiley, New York.

Landsbergis, P.A. (1988) Occupational stress among health care workers: a test of the job demands-control model. *Journal of Organisational Behaviour*, **9**, 217–39.

McGrath, J.E. (1976) Stress and behaviour in organisations, in Dunnette, M.D. (ed.) *Handbook of Industrial and Organisational Psychology*, John Wiley, New York.

McLean, A.A. (1980) *Work Stress*, Addison-Wiley, Reading, Massachusetts.

Margolis, B., Kroes, W. and Quinn, R. (1974) Job stress an unlisted 'occupational' hazard. *Journal of Occupational Medicine*, **1**(16), 659–61.

Maslach, C. (1982a) Understanding burnout: definitional issues in analysing a complex phenomenon, in Paine, W.S. (ed.) *Job Stress and*

Burnout: Research Theory and Intervention Perspectives, Sage, Beverly Hills.

Maslach, C. (1982b) *Burnout – The Cost of Coping*, Prentice Hall, Hemel Hempstead.

Mavtocchio, J.J. and O'Leary, A.M. (1989) Sex differences in occupational stress: a meta-analytic review. *Journal of American Psychology*, **74**, 495–501.

Miles, R.H. and Perrault, W.D. (1976) Organisational role conflicts: job antecendants and consequences. *Organisational Behaviour and Human Performance*, **17**, 19–44.

Miner, J.B. and Brewer, J.F. (1976) Management of ineffective performance, in Dunnette, M.D. (ed.) *Handbook of Industrial and Organisational Psychology*, Rand McNally, Chicago.

Newton, T.J. (1989) Occupational stress and coping with stress: a critique. *Human Relations*, **42**(5), 441–61.

Osipow, S.H., Doty, R.E., and Spokame, A.R. (1985) Occupational stress, strain and coping across the life span. *Journal of Vocational Behaviour*, **27**(1), 98–108.

Paffenbarger, R.S., Wolf, P.A. and Notkin, J. (1966) Chronic disease in former college students. *American Journal of Epidemiology*, **83**, 314–28.

Parlmore, E. (1969) Predicting longevity: a follow-up controlling for age. *The Gerontologist*, **9**, 247–50.

Payne, R. (1988) Individual differences in the study of occupational stress, in Cooper, C.L. and Payne, R. (eds) *Causes, Coping and Consequences of Stress at Work*, John Wiley, Chichester.

Perrewe, P.L. and Ganster, P.C. (1989) The impact of job demands and behaviourial control on experienced job stress. *Journal of Occupational Behaviour*, **10**, 213–29.

Quick, J.C. and Quick, J.D. (1984) *Organisational Stress and Preventive Management*, Mcgraw Hill, New York.

Quinn, R.P. and Staines, G.L. (1979) *The 1977 Quality of Employment Survey*, Institute for Social Research, Ann Arbor.

Reich, S. and Geller, A. (1976a) Self image of nurses. Psychological Report, October, 401–2.

Reich, S. and Geller, A. (1976b) Self image of social workers. Psychological Report, October, 657–8.

Roos, P.E. and Cohen, L.H. (1987) Social roles and social support as moderators of life stress and adjustment. *Journal of Personal and Social Psychology*, **52**, 576–85.

Rutenfranz, J., Colquhoun, W., Knauth, P. and Ghata, J. (1974) Biomedical and psychosocial aspects of shift work. *Scandinavian Journal of Work Environment and Health*, **3**, 165–82.

Selye, H. (1976) *The Stress of Life*, McGraw Hill, New York.

Singer, G. (1985) New approaches to social factors in shiftwork, in Wallace, M. (ed.) *Shiftwork and Health*, Brain Behaviour Research Institute, Bundora, Australia.

Smith, M.J., Cohen, R.G., Stammerjohn, L.W. and Happ, A. (1981) An investigation of health complaints and job stress in video display operations. *Human Factors*, **23**, 389–400.

Smith, M.J., Colligan, M.J., and Tasto, D.L. (1982) Health and safety consequences of shift work in the food processing industry. *Ergonomics*, **25**, 133–44.

Steers, R.M. and Rhodes, S.R. (1978) Major influences on employee attendance: a process model. *Journal of Applied Psychology*, **63**, 391–407.

Super, D.E., Stariskevsky, R., Matlin, N. and Jordaan, J.P. (1963) *Career Development: Self Concept Theory*, College Entrance Examinations Board, New York.

Sutherland, V.J. (1990) Managing stress at the worksite, in Bennett, P., Weinman, J. and Spurgeon, P. (eds) *Current Developments in Health Psychology*, Harwood Academic Press, London.

Sutherland, V.J. and Cooper, C.L. (1986) *Man and Accidents Offshore: The Costs of Stress Among Workers on Oil and Gas Rigs*, Lloyd's List/Detsman (International) NV, London.

Sutherland, V.J. and Cooper, C.L. (1988) Sources of work stress, in Hurrell, J.J. Jr., Murphy, L.R., Sauter, S.L. and Cooper, C.L. (eds) *Occupational Stress: Issues and Developments in Research*, Taylor & Francis, London.

Sutherland, V.J. and Cooper, C.L. (1992) Job stress, satisfaction and mental health among general practitioners before and after the introduction of new contracts. *British Medical Journal*, **304**, 1545–8.

Thomas, C.B. and Duszynski, K.R. (1974) Closeness to parents and the family constellation in a prospective study of five disease states: suicide, mental illness, malignant tumour, hypertension and coronary heart disease. *John Hopkins Medical Journal*, **134**, 251–70.

Waldgrave, W. (1992) Introduction in Jenkins, R. and Coney, N., *Prevention of Mental Ill Health at Work*, HMSO, London.

Warr, P. and Wall, T. (1975) *Work and Well-being*, Penguin Books, Harmondsworth.

World Health Organisation (1986) *Constitution of the World Health Organisation*, in Basic Documents – 36th edition.

6

Health promotion in the workplace

Jane Molloy

INTRODUCTION

The philosophical basis of occupational health (OH) lies in its commitment to a two-pronged strategy: to the protection of the worker from illness or injury arising as a result of work activity and to the promotion of health and well-being by the provision of strategies that encompass occupational, lifestyle, environmental, political, social and legal factors and emphasize self-empowered decision-making.

Occupational health nursing is a highly specialized, albeit small, branch of nursing within which the OH nurse is frequently required to work as a member of a multi-disciplinary team. Although founded on the traditional nursing role, the knowledge base of OH nursing draws on a number of diverse disciplines. Among other things, the practice of OH nursing embraces health education, disease prevention and health protection which, according to Andrew Tannahill, formerly Senior Lecturer in Public Health Medicine, University of Glasgow, comprise the essential elements of a model of health promotion and which help in 'defining, planning and "doing" health promotion' (Downie, Fyfe and Tannahill, 1990: 57).

The multi-disciplinary team in occupational health practice involves professionals who share a common knowledge. The OH team in an organization may be comprised of disciplines such as medicine, nursing, management, occupational hygiene, toxicology, epidemiology, ergonomics, occupational psychology and safety.

When discussing a conceptual model for OH nursing practice in 1985, Linda Morris suggested that co-operation within the team in regard to problem-solving is essential if occupationally related illness is to be prevented and the concept of a team approach to promoting health in the workplace is a distinct and desirable possibility. This view is endorsed by Molle and Allan (1989) who believe that OH nurses, along with other professionals, are in a good position to alter the emphasis and direction of health care. They go on to highlight the need for OH nurses to work with others:

> to develop programs that are cost-effective, scientifically sound and based on documented health needs and health values of workers.
>
> (Molle and Allan, 1989, p. 522)

They also suggest that in many organizations the OH nurse may be the only health-care professional and may need to work closely with management in developing health-promotion programmes.

The promotion of health in the workplace is not a new concept and can be traced back to the early eighteenth century. Shephard (1986) quotes Ramazzini (1713):

> It is a laughable sight to see these guilds of cobblers and tailors . . . a troop of stooping, round-shouldered, limping men, swaying from side to side . . . they should be advised to take physical exercise at any rate on holidays.

Two centuries later, the first medical inspector of factories, Sir Thomas Legge (1934, p. 3) stated:

> all the workmen should be told something of the danger of the material with which they come into contact and not be left to find out for themselves – sometimes at the cost of their lives.

Although radical thinkers like Ramazzini and Legge were clearly aware of the need for health-promotion strategies at work, there are many employers today who persist in intransigent attitudes towards the promotion of the health of employees. Watterson

(1986, p. 77) identifies three ways in which the idea of worker protection against workplace health risks is challenged by employers:

1. Britain's health and safety at work record is excellent. We have few accidents and even fewer diseases.
2. Jobs are crucial to the economy and if we want employment we must risk a few accidents and illnesses at work.
3. Where accidents do occur at work careless and stupid workers are to blame.

However, Schilling (1989) suggests that many occupational health services in larger organizations in the United Kingdom do engage in health-promotion programmes for their employees. This was endorsed by the findings of the IRS Employment Trends survey (1989) which suggested that the workplace is now being recognized as a valuable forum for initiatives designed to promote the health and fitness of employees. This survey of health promotion activities in 50 organizations showed a marked increase in the number of employers who have initiated health-promotion activities in recent years.

According to Popp (1989) the enhancement of health among the workforce must be viewed in the context of responsibility shared between employer and worker since, for occupational-health strategies to be successful, workers must be educated to understand that their health is something for which they too are responsible (Popp, 1989). Such education requires professionally trained occupational health staff, such as occupational-health nurses, who are well-placed to carry out education and health promotion activities and to plan, develop, implement and evaluate worksite health-promotion programmes.

In the USA in the last 10 to 15 years, many corporate organizations have revolutionized their attitudes towards the health of employees (Ashton, 1989), and workplace health-promotion programmes appear to be flourishing. Attitudes in the UK, it seems, are less enthusiastic, not least because of a lack of funding for health-promotion activities. For example, of the £26 billion currently spent on the National Health Service (NHS), only £20 million were allocated to the Health Education Authority. This represents a mere 0.07% of total spending on health (Ashton, 1989).

Many would argue a lack of supporting scientific data regarding the benefit of workplace health-promotion activities and that those who do advocate such programmes base their reasons on anecdotal evidence only. However, as Ashton (1989) rightly points out, it does not follow that health-promotion programmes are of no benefit simply because scientific studies to prove their worth have not been undertaken.

Others would argue that programmes designed to address lifestyle-risk factors do not fall within the remit of workplace-health provision. But the fact that many people spend approximately a third of their lives in a work setting would seem to suggest that the working environment should embrace the health of the individual in all its facets.

Gordon (1987) considers the social and political context in which workplace-health promotion takes place to be worthy of serious attention and that such programmes should emphasize a holistic approach towards health. Therefore, in her view, it is necessary to consider aspects such as economic status, individual lifestyle, home and work stress, heredity factors and existing health problems as well as health associated with occupational factors.

Ashton (1989, p. 27), referring to health-promotion activities in the UK, states:

> organisations, together with occupational health physicians and nurses, are in a unique position to influence the health of the workforce of this country.

Certainly the use of the workplace as a setting for health-promotion programmes gives the health promoter access to a 'captive' audience, to a large proportion of the healthy adult population and to established lines of communication. Ashton (1989) believes that the issue of health promotion for workers currently present occupational-health professionals with a challenge and opportunity which they cannot, or should not, ignore.

The purpose of this chapter is to examine the present provision of workplace-health promotion; to clarify the role of the OH nurse; to identify the potential benefits and pitfalls of a team approach to promoting health at work; and to identify current research in the field.

PROVISION OF HEALTH PROMOTION IN THE WORKPLACE

Although Britain has a population in excess of 55 million of which 28 million are members of the workforce, the main focus of health care has tended towards primary care in the community (Webb *et al.*, 1988). The working population of Britain is comprised mainly of 'healthy' adults and this section will seek to examine the extent to which health-promoting activities are provided for this population.

Occupational health services were originally designed to provide treatment for those employees who become ill or injured at work. The emphasis was on the restorative nature of nursing and medicine and little attention was given to the protection of workers, the prevention of ill health and injury, or the promotion of health. However, the last ten years have seen a growing awareness, both in the UK and the USA, of the need for preventive strategies and the workplace is now concerning itself more with both occupational and general health issues.

Referring to the situation in the USA, Fielding (1990) suggests there are several reasons for the recent growth in workplace health-promotion programmes and includes the growing evidence to link worker health and productivity with the rapidly escalating health care benefit payments for employees borne by employers. Twenty years ago the cost of health care in the USA was considered by employers to be a minor expense (Whitmer cited in Selleck *et al.* 1989) but today rising employee costs are a problem of great magnitude. This has resulted in the emergence of employee health-promotion programmes based on the rationale that it costs less to educate workers about controllable health risks than to pay for the cost of ill health (Brennan, 1983).

Christenson and Kiefhaber (1988) suggest that the national trend toward the promotion of health at work has been encouraged by employers' increased attention to health issues, and to employees' desire to work in a healthy environment. In the USA national interest in health-related behaviour, such as exercise, weight control and so on, began with the recognition that the leading causes of death had shifted from communicable to chronic diseases. According to the IRS (1989) survey, a similar picture is emerging in the UK where in recent years there has been a marked increase in the number of organizations that have initiated health-promotion activities.

A major difference between the UK and the USA appears to be the area of accountability for health-care costs. In the USA such costs are borne either by the individual or, more commonly, by the employer, while in the UK costs are mostly the responsibility of the whole community. However, with the advent of the British government's 1986 Social Security Act and the placement of responsibility for statutory sick pay on the shoulders of employers, this position appears to be changing and could account for the sharp increase in health-promotion activities since 1986 as cited in the IRS (1989) survey.

In the USA, 1985 saw the first national survey of worksite health-promotion activities, the results of which were reported in 1988. The objectives of the survey were to:

- determine the nature and extent of health-promotion activities in worksites of 50 or more employees;
- determine what employers perceive as the direct and indirect benefits of their efforts to prevent disease and promote employee health;
- monitor progress toward the worksite health-promotion goals set forth in the '1990 Health Promotion Objectives for the Nation'.

(Christenson and Kiefhaber, 1988, p. 262)

The findings of the national survey indicated that improved employee health was the most frequently cited reason for offering a health-promotion activity and this finding was consistent with earlier research. Towers (1984, cited in Eriksen, 1988), commenting on a 1983 survey, states that 60% of both employers and union leaders believe 'wellness' programmes to be useful in improving overall employee health. Although this latter finding is encouraging, the fact remains that 40% of employers and union leaders did not endorse this view.

Prior to the national survey, *The Surgeon General's Report on Health Promotion and Disease Prevention* (1979) identified the worksite as an appropriate milieu for health promotion and it is possible that this has encouraged and stimulated the acceptance of worksite health promotion by employers.

In the UK, progress has been somewhat slower but a major survey was undertaken by the Health Education Council in 1986 which sought to identify occupational health-promotion developments in the last ten years and to highlight issues which future health promotion activists should address. In particular, the researchers explored the potential paths of development for occupational health services and these are summarized below:

- the extent to which such occupational health services can, and should, be involved in the prevention of workplace hazards;
- the extent to which this work should be concerned, not merely with the hazards that may have their origins in the workplace directly, but in promoting changes that can benefit the health of employees, their families and even the community generally;
- the influences that have shaped developments in the past ten years and the resources that might best help future developments.

(Webb *et al.*, 1988, p. 15)

The researchers collected their data from major employers and employers' associations, trade unions and organizations with an interest in workplace health promotion. The results of the survey showed marked differences between the views of employers' associations and trade unions. For example, 70% of trade unions had developed policies on health promotion compared to 60% of public sector employers and only 20% of large private sector employers. The data collected about occupational health issues and health-promotion programme activities also showed some differences, notably that trade unions had given higher priority to reproductive hazards to employees than had employers' associations. When considering the future, the researchers believe that the findings reveal the possibility of small but significant shifts in emphasis:

- it is noticable that alcohol, stress and nutrition programmes now equal or out-number programmes on the traditional occupational health issues of safety, noise and dusts;
- other health promotion programmes such as smoking and screening are being planned.

(Webb *et al.*, 1988, p. 17)

The researchers warn that it would be easy to infer too much from the findings of this report. Indeed, the questionnaire responses to 'programme activity' are open to wide interpretation by respondents. However, when issues were put into order of priority, the researchers identified a definite pattern and hazards relating to smoking, alcohol and stress were seen to be issues of as great importance as those of noise and dust. Reproductive hazards and nutrition were also considered to be significant issues.

When attempting to translate the priorities identified into practical health policies, the researchers caution about the possibility of employers misusing the results of the survey by adopting a 'victim-blaming' attitude. For example, as a result of the study employers may exhort workers to change their lifestyles and at the same time use this as an opportunity to ignore changes in working practices and policy.

In the USA, 2.5 million people are disabled by occupational accidents and diseases each year (Crawford, 1977). Management in corporate organizations are increasingly blaming the workforce, and in particular the individual worker, by suggesting that of the large number of accidental deaths at work, most are caused by worker carelessness, laziness about wearing protective equipment, psychological maladjustment or worker susceptibility to ill health (Crawford, 1977). A further concern voiced by Crawford is that managements in the USA appear to be integrating victim-blaming themes into their personnel policies. He suggests that:

> Holding individual workers responsible for their susceptibility to illness . . . reinforces management attempts to control absenteeism and enhance productivity.
>
> (Crawford, 1977, p. 673)

Writing as long ago as 1977, Crawford's views are as pertinent today as they were then and the implications of such thinking are far-reaching. If workers are seen by management not to be paying sufficient attention to their health, then it is a short step to sanctions, dismissals or early retirement.

The importance of the HEC study (Webb *et al.*, 1988) and its implications for occupational health practice should not be understated and the researchers warn that although fairly substantial progress with regard to developing an agenda for health promotion and ill health prevention has been achieved in the last ten years, there is no room for complacency and there is still a long way to go in approaching the goals of the WHO *Health For All by the Year 2000* campaign. Indeed, their goals are more ambitious and they state that:

we need to overcome the inertia that is inhibiting the development of workplace health for the vast majority of British workers and workplaces.

(Webb *et al.*, 1988, p. 35)

Webb *et al.* (1988) expound their belief that it would be impossible for community-based health services to cope with the special needs and problems of the workplace:

In many cases the community health professionals have neither the skills nor the training necessary for preventive work.

(Webb *et al.*, 1988, p. 36)

They go on to recommend that the skills of workplace health professionals 'such as occupational health nurses and nurse practitioners' (p. 36) should be utilized more fully and they advocate a team approach in order to provide for smaller organizations. Smogor and Macrina (1987) refer to the plight of small organizations in the USA, suggesting that little research has been done on the nature of, or need for, health-promotion programmes in small businesses, the employees of which often make up the majority of the total labour force in the USA. Fielding and Breslow's (1983) survey of perceptions of health promotion by small businesses found that employers considered health-promotion programmes to be unneccessary: 'no need exists because employees are healthy' (p. 225). Perhaps the perpetuation of this attitude is the consequence of a society which, for many years, has mainly emphasized the 'acute' aspects of health care.

Fielding (1990) believes economic return to be the strongest argument to influence American employers to implement health-promotion strategies at the workplace. He cites the 'Johnson and Johnson' comparative study which identified the relationship between exposure to a worksite health-promotion programme, *Live for Life*, and employer-borne health-care costs. The results suggest a positive impact both on the utilization of health services and on health-care costs.

In the UK, the IRS Employment Trends (1989) study of the health-promotion activities of 50 organizations highlights employers' references to health-promotion activities as proving a help in reducing the levels of sickness absence. However, the organizations surveyed in this study were selected from subscribers to occupational health-and-safety specialist journals and may not, therefore, be representative of organizations generally. However, despite its limitations, the study is important because it highlights those health issues employers consider most important (Table 6.1).

Table 6.1 League table of health priorities

Health promotion issues	Average score	'Top priority' scores	'Lowest priority' score
Smoking	2.02	28	7
Cervical screening	2.41	13	4
Stress	2.42	17	8
Breast screening	2.44	12	3
Alcohol/drugs	2.48	16	5
Fitness/exercise	2.56	5	
Nutrition	2.79	10	8
Health/welfare advice	2.83	9	7
Obesity control	2.89	8	10
Personal development	3.00	9	9
Sex-related diseases	3.15	7	10
Antenatal care	3.43	9	15
Maternity care	3.52	9	19
Contraception	3.60	7	20

Source: IRS Employment Trends 443, p. 13.

Schilling (1989) refers to the government's plans to encourage health-promoting strategies and activities among family doctors and primary health-care teams in the UK, and highlights the fact that occupational health services have been excluded. He goes on to enumerate the reasons he believes health promotion should be provided in workplaces:

1. occupational health services have ready access to people before they get sick;
2. economic benefits to the employer should follow the reduction of unnecessary disability and the promotion of better health.

(Schilling, 1989, p. 686)

But he cautions that to be accepted, good evidence of the effectiveness of co-ordinated health-promotion programmes in British workplaces is needed. Such evidence can only be obtained if health promoters evaluate their activities, and such evaluation, it seems, both in the USA and the UK, is seriously lacking.

According to Fielding (1990) most employers lack interest or expertise in undertaking an evaluation which would be acceptable to academic scrutiny. He suggests that most benefits of health-promotion activities are determined by anecdotal reporting. However, on a more optimistic note, he suggests that university researchers are becoming increasingly involved in the formal evaluation of worksite health-promotion programmes in the USA and he continues:

> published results of evaluations to date suggest that worksite health promotion programs can have positive impacts on health behaviours and health status.
>
> (Fielding, 1990, p. 75)

Alternatively evaluation is, or perhaps should be, part of the work of a skilled occupational health nurse. The following section will attempt to identify the literature relating to the role of the OH nurse in health promotion.

PROMOTING HEALTH IN OH NURSING PRACTICE

Since the late-nineteenth century, occupational health nursing practice has changed considerably from a curative 'medical' model to one in which the main focus is the prevention of ill health, accident and injury and the promotion of health and well-being. This transition from a 'curative' to a 'preventive' model has happened gradually, but the last ten years has seen an escalation in the health-promotion activities of OH nurses in the UK. Many, it seems, have embraced and developed the role of health promoter voluntarily; others have become involved in order to comply with the philosophy of the organization for which they are working.

Historically, OH nurses have been the recipients of specialized education which has aimed to prepare them for their role in disease prevention and health promotion. Archer (1983), in a study of the impact of continuing education on OH nursing practice, investigated the relationship between continuing education and the quality of health-promotion programmes offered to employees by OH nurses. The findings of the study suggest a significant relationship between the number of years in OH nursing practice and programme planning and implementation. Archer concludes that those OH nurses who have received more specialized OH nursing education are more likely to be offering a greater range of disease prevention and health-promotion programmes.

Popp (1989, p. 114) refers to the OH nurse as being one of a range of professionals who are currently 'learning about health promotion and see it as an arena for their skills'. Taylor (1987, p. 114) believes that OH nurses should capitalize on the present climate. She maintains that OH nurses are in a unique position to:

> identify and influence the action of management in the areas of lifestyle, health perceptions and attitudes, and organisational efforts to promote health.

Among other things, this requires an ability to advise management about funding priorities for health-promotion activities as well as the potential cost effectiveness of such activities.

Taylor (1987) reports how an OH nurse, working in a one-nurse unit, successfully implemented a major workplace health-promotion programme. However, to achieve success any such programme must have the approval and active participation of management, for without this a programme will be doomed to failure. In Taylor's study the skills used to gain management's approval and financial support were essential and she describes her strategy which involved a comprehensive presentation to management to demonstrate the cost-effectiveness of the programme. She used a three-pronged approach:

- reduction of health-care costs;
- reduced absenteeism;
- analysis of cost effectiveness.

Popp (1989) identifies the importance of OH nurses anticipating and addressing the ethical issues involved in health promotion and suggests that these be considered at the planning stage of the programme proposing review of:

- paternalistic attitude of the company;
- job discrimination on the basis of poor health;
- differences in 'white collar' and 'blue collar' workers' access to health promotion activities.

Further to the latter point, a study carried out by Schenck *et al.*

(1987) investigated such differences among rubber workers. The study examined workplace health policy and lifestyle health promotion. Findings indicate that workers showed a strong interest in receiving more programmes relating both to health protection and health promotion and that 94% of the blue collar workers expressed an interest in stress management, contrary to popular belief that this is more the concern of white collar workers.

Gott and O'Brien (1989) investigated the role of the nurse in the UK in health promotion. They explored nurses' roles in different settings, namely community, general and occupational health nursing. The study suggested certain ethical issues to be specific to OH nursing practice, in particular the area of accountability, for example, to employee, employer or to the nursing profession?

In Gott and O'Brien's study, both OH nurses and health visitors perceived health promotion to be an important part of their role. However, they found that many nurses appear to be unaware of local health-promotion plans and few are involved in policy planning. The researchers go on to discuss the role of the nurse in facilitating client access to health services and suggest that such facilitation is dependent on the nurse's ability to mobilize resources from various organizations, including the one in which they are employed. The study highlights several factors that Gott and O'Brien believe to be crucial if nurses are properly to embrace a health-promoting strategy in their work:

- the way in which nurses encounter the health-seeking public – this involves the relationships between nurses and 'clients' and the settings in which the encounters take place;
- the ability of nurses to formulate for health organisations the needs and desires of clients;
- the manner in which knowledge about health and health resources is conveyed to clients and the manner in which such knowledge is conveyed to nurses;
- the ways that nurses together with other health agents frame their actions in order to achieve consistent health promoting behaviours and initiatives.

(Gott and O'Brien, 1989, p. 18)

The results of Gott and O'Brien's study indicate the importance of the work-setting in influencing both the range of nurses' activities and the extent of their professional relationships within the organization. For example, one OH department of an NHS hospital offered a general screening service to hospital workers. The researchers report that although OH nurses attempted to assess clients' knowledge of lifestyle health risks and corrected any misconceptions, the activity emphasized individual behaviour change and did not address the wider social and economic issues. This was in marked contrast to one of the industrial settings investigated where the OH nurse was well-supported by management:

> given time, resources and training to get the workforce involved in making decisions about a company smoking policy, organising committees on health and safety, drafting and monitoring welfare services suited to the changing size and activities of the company.
>
> (Gott and O'Brien, 1989, p. 30)

Such an environment enabled the OH nurse to represent to senior management the needs and desires of the workers. However, she acknowledged that cartain environmental constraints are inevitable and accepted that the productivity of the company will be its first priority. Gott and O'Brien (1989) believe that such conditions have the potential to raise moral and ethical issues for OH nurses.

In the same study Gott and O'Brien investigated ways in which nurses acquire both their knowledge about health and the skills needed for health-promotion activities. Findings related to the latter indicate many nurses' feelings of not having received training for many of the skills needed for health-promotion activities. The researchers found that all nurses considered continued learning to be very important and frequently named constant change in the requirements of their work as a reason to continue this process. The researchers' overall impression was:

> What knowledge they (the participants) had about health promotion had been acquired by themselves and not as a result of teaching or instruction.

The results of Gott and O'Brien's work are the preliminary findings of a pilot study; they refer to a small sample and cannot be generalized to the wider population. But the issues raised are interesting and worthy of consideration.

In a study to determine the extent to which the health education component of the OH nursing course meets the needs of practising OH nurses, Molloy (1990) found that some employers actively encouraged and expected OH nurses to carry out workplace health-promotion programmes as a major part of their role. One participant indicated that her employer not only supported such initiatives, but positively expected the OH nurse to spend approximately 50% of her time planning, implementing and evaluating workplace health-promotion programmes.

In the same study, which involved a small sample of participants, all those interviewed considered health-promotion activities to be an important part of the job. A similar finding was reported by Gott and O'Brien (1989) in their investigation of work role and perceptions of health promotion among health visitors and OH nurses. In Molloy's (1990) study the majority of respondents indicated that they undertake health-education programmes on a regular basis; but this finding should be interpreted with caution since both the size and the method of selecting the sample introduced potential biases into the study.

As previously suggested, the philosophy underpinning OH nursing lies in its commitment to worker health and well-being through strategies designed to prevent the occurrence of ill-health, to educate for and about health, and to promote health both individually and collectively. The fulfilment of these aims requires a comprehensive approach to health promotion and a method by which this can be achieved is that of teamworking.

TEAMWORK

A team approach to promoting health is advocated by Ewles and Simnett (1992) who suggest that health promotion frequently involves different disciplines working together which necessarily requires good co-ordination and teamwork. They identify certain characteristics which may be applied to a successful team:

- a team consists of a group of identified people;
- the team has a common purpose and shared objectives which are known and agreed by all members;
- the team has a leader whose authority is accepted by all members;

- team members are selected because they have relevant expertise;
- members know and agree their own role and know the roles of the other members;
- members support each other in achieving their common purpose;
- members trust each other, and communicate with each other in an open, honest way.

(Ewles and Simnett, 1992, p. 106)

Teamwork in occupational health involves professionals who share a core of knowledge. The composition of the OH team will necessarily differ according to the needs of the organization, but the common goal is to provide care and to protect the health of the worker from any harmful agent – physical, chemical, biological or psychosocial. Such protection of health and enhancement of well-being necessarily involves the formulation of health-promotion strategies for the workforce. But irrespective of the number of specialists employed in a single team, members will always work more effectively if they understand each others' roles, aims and objectives, and accept that roles will inevitably overlap. It follows, then, that an essential requirement for the OH nurse is that they should understand the principles underlying the disciplines of team members.

In the OH setting, each team member should be able to provide specific skills which are unique to their discipline while the common goal of all members of the OH team is to ensure a healthy workforce. However, it has been suggested that, in practice, problems of teamwork may reveal animosity, role conflict, poor communication and concerns with leadership status (Hunt, 1974; Bowling, 1983). This is endorsed by Ross (1987) who warns that there are many barriers to teamwork such as the unequal balance of power between professionals and the client (or worker). She also suggests that teamwork may have the negative effect of concealing differences in knowledge and expectations between individual professionals. However, in her investigation of the primary health-care team, Ross (1987) identifies some common characteristics of an integrated team:

- a common purpose;
- shared decision-making;
- overlapping roles;

- shifting leadership focus;
- willingness of team members to subordinate their own interests to the shared interest of the group.

These characteristics bear resemblance to those identified by Ewles and Simnett (1992) with the exception of the role of leader; and it would seem wise for OH team members to give consideration to these characteristics if involved in an interdisciplinary approach to the planning, implementation and evaluation of health-promotion programmes for the workforce.

It is now generally accepted by health professionals that the word 'health' has a range of different meanings and from this it can be deduced that for successful health promotion to occur a variety of strategies need to be considered. The following section will seek to provide a framework for OH nursing practice which is flexible enough to embrace the different health-promotion approaches deemed necessary for promoting health in an occupational-health environment.

APPLICATION TO PRACTISE

Before embarking on the practicalities of workplace health promotion, it is worth considering, albeit briefly, the question 'Why occupational health nurses?' If it is accepted that neither health nor health promotion are the sole property of health professionals and, as Seedhouse (1986) argues, that health should be viewed as 'a universal concern' and therefore the business of everyone, why then should health promotion be a major role of the practising occupational health nurse?

One of the key objectives of OH nursing practice is that nurses should take a leading role in preventing ill health and promoting well-being and so act as promoters of health. By virtue of their training and specialist education they are well-placed to carry out this role which is viewed by the Royal College of Nursing as one of the main routes to professional excellence.

The government's White Paper *The Health of the Nation* (1992) identifies among its aims the need to provide tangible goals to improve health, with an emphasis on prevention. Sadly, the contribution of OH practitioners in realizing the achievement of these aims appears to have been disregarded in this document.

In common with other fields of nursing, the benefits of occupational health promotion are many and include advantages for both the employer and the worker. For example, a study carried out among Finnish farmers (Vohlonen *et al.*, 1985, cited in Radford 1990) showed an increase in the use of personal safety devices as a direct result of OH nurses providing education on this issue. Another Finnish study in which the OH nurse played a prominent part was that of Frilander *et al.* (1986) cited in Radford (1990), whose findings suggest that the use of health-promotion strategies resulted in a reduction in absenteeism. The findings of Blair *et al.*'s (1986) large-scale study (cited in Tones, Tilford and Robinson, 1990) also identified significant reduction in absenteeism. Specific benefits to the worker include:

- an increase in knowledge relevant to the prevention of occupational injury and disease and the promotion of health and well-being;
- an increase in morale as a result of involvement in decision-making;
- changes in occupational health policy as a result of OH nurses involvement in research devoted to the promotion of health at work.

Having established the need for OH nurses to take a key role in workplace health-promotion activities, a framework proposed by Ewles and Simnett (1992) will next be examined.

A FRAMEWORK FOR PRACTICE

The framework for health-promotion activities devised by Ewles and Simnett (1992) (Fig. 6.1) provides a useful model to help clarify the activities with which the health promoter may be involved.

It is not the intention of Ewles and Simnett that the framework should be viewed as a rigid classification. Indeed, they are at pains to point out that activities may not always fall neatly into the identified categories and that overlap will inevitably occur. They also state clearly that the framework cannot encompass the entire gamut of activities and that some health promotion will occur both informally and incidentally. Of great importance, according to the authors, is that health promoters should become aware that health promotion embraces a wide range of activities.

The framework comprises seven clear areas of health pro-

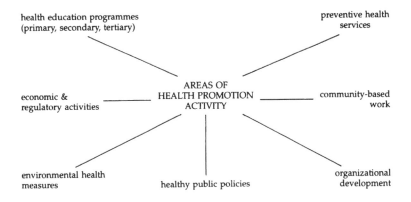

Figure 6.1 A framework for health-promotion activities. (Source: Ewles, L. and Simnett, I. (1992) *Promoting Health: A Practical Guide*).

motion activity (Fig. 6.1) and is concerned with 'planned, deliberate activities' (p. 26). Each of the seven areas will be considered individually and suggestions made as to how such a framework can be applied to an occupational-health environment (Fig. 6.2).

HEALTH EDUCATION PROGRAMMES

The majority of workplace health-education programmes fall into the category of primary-health education: i.e. education directed at 'healthy' people. Examples of such education include:

a) *general lifestyle*
   healthy eating
   fitness/exercise
   smoking/alcohol
   womens'/mens' health
   sexual health

b) *work-related topics*
   food hygiene
   lifting and handling
   work stress
   hearing conservation
   HIV/AIDS and the workplace

However, it is unrealistic to expect that members of the working population will always be at an optimum state of health and strategies for both secondary and tertiary health education are required. For example, the OH nurse may adopt the role of facilitator of a 'Sensible Drinking' group set up specifically to help those for whom excessive consumption of alcohol has

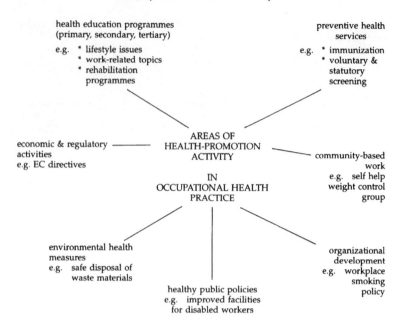

health education programmes
(primary, secondary, tertiary)

e.g. * lifestyle issues
     * work-related topics
     * rehabilitation
       programmes

preventive health
services

e.g. * immunization
     * voluntary &
       statutory
       screening

economic & regulatory
activities
e.g. EC directives

AREAS OF
HEALTH-PROMOTION
ACTIVITY

community-based
work
e.g.   self help
weight control
group

IN
OCCUPATIONAL HEALTH
PRACTICE

environmental health
measures
e.g.   safe disposal of
       waste materials

organizational
development
e.g. workplace
smoking
policy

healthy public policies
e.g. improved facilities
      for disabled workers

Figure 6.2 Application of Ewles and Simnett (1992) framework for health-promotion activities to occupational health practice.

become a contributory factor toward their present state of ill health (i.e. secondary education); or the OH nurse may provide help and support in the rehabilitation of a worker who has suffered a traumatic accident resulting in amputation of a limb (i.e. tertiary education).

PREVENTIVE HEALTH SERVICES

A prime function of occupational-health practice is the provision of preventive health services. The type of services offered is variable and depends on the size and nature of the industry as well as the philosophy of the organization. But it is likely that the majority of employers provide both voluntary and statutory health screening and many offer immunization programmes.

COMMUNITY-BASED WORK

The workplace provides an opportunity for people to engage in self-help activities. Such activities are 'worker led': the workers identify their own health needs and actively participate in addressing them. An example could be a group of workers who have concerns about their weight and who set up their own workplace 'weight watchers' group, facilitated by the occupational health nurse.

ORGANIZATIONAL DEVELOPMENT

According to Tones, Tilford and Robinson (1990), in recent years policy development in workplaces has tended to focus on alcohol, smoking, fitness and nutrition. Many employers, for example, now make reference to a 'No Smoking' policy when advertising for new recruits.

HEALTHY PUBLIC POLICY

Occupational health practitioners are well-placed to influence management about policies that may affect the wider population, for example, policies aimed at improving and increasing facilities for disabled people at work.

ENVIRONMENTAL HEALTH MEASURES

In recent years environmental issues have been high on the agenda of OH professionals, not only in relation to improved physical conditions for the workforce, but also in respect of the effect of workplace activities on the health and well-being of the community at large. For example, efforts to ensure the safe disposal of waste materials may provide protection not only for those within the working environment but also for the surrounding community.

ECONOMIC AND REGULATORY ACTIVITIES

Since the nineteenth century, government legislation has attempted to provide safeguards in respect of workplace activities. The 1974 Health and Safety at Work Act emphasized the need for both employer and employee to accept responsibility in regard to health and safety and to recognize the importance of participation in pursuit of its achievement. More recently, an immense increase in new legislative measures, largely in response to the rapid introduction of European Community (EC) Directives concerning health and safety, has been evident. However, co-operation is essential if legislation is to be successful as a measure of health protection.

In summary, it seems that the framework for health-promotion activities can be used to guide the health-promotion work of practising OH nurses and is a useful reminder that such work covers a broad range of activities. But as well as recognizing the areas of health-promotion activity, OH nurses need to acquire and develop skills and abilities which will enable them to put their knowledge of health promotion into practice.

SKILLS AND ABILITIES

Organizing and managing a workplace health-promotion programme can be time-consuming and necessarily requires careful and painstaking planning. There are certain key steps which are worth considering.

Reviewing needs and priorities

When contemplating workplace health promotion, Tones, Tilford and Robinson (1990) suggest there are two conflicting interests that govern the frequently disparate needs of those concerned:

1. Management needs:
   those for whom the profit motive is the major concern;
2. Health promoter needs:
   those for whom the enhancement of well-being may be the prime objective.

The needs of the workers, it is suggested, will probably fall somewhere between 1. and 2. (Tones, Tilford and Robinson, 1990). If this is the case, then any assessment of priorities will necessarily involve due consideration of three domains of need (Fig. 6.3).

The adoption of an epidemiological approach is one method

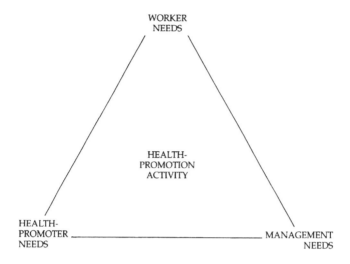

WORKER
NEEDS

HEALTH-
PROMOTION
ACTIVITY

HEALTH-
PROMOTER
NEEDS

MANAGEMENT
NEEDS

Figure 6.3   Three domains of perceived need.

by which workplace needs and priorities can be determined. Such an approach raises important questions:

- is there a need?
- how serious is the need?
- is it amenable to health promotion?
- can the costs of a programme be justified?
- would a programme be ethically acceptable?

Application of these questions may reveal a range of occupational health-promotion needs deserving attention. But one of the skills of the health promoter is the ability to rank such needs in relation to the availability of time, energy and resources.

Closely associated with the ability to review needs and priorities is the ability to undertake a realistic assessment of the scope and limitations of the proposed health-promotion activity.

ASSESSMENT

The ability to undertake a comprehensive assessment is a necessary prerequisite of all health professionals and the occupational health promoter is no exception. Health promotion is, or should be, a two-way process: a learning experience shared between the person promoting health and well-being and the 'learners'. Thus assessment of the intended target group or individual is of paramount importance if appropriate and relevant health promotion is to be ensured.

Such an assessment may involve collecting information about the group itself – for example, age/sex/existing level of knowledge – so as to identify specific needs and appropriate health-promotion strategies. The support and co-operation of both the workforce and management is essential if successful health promotion is to occur. Thus the involvement of both in the decision-making process when examining and selecting appropriate options should help to secure this needed support as well as to guard against decisions being solely professionally defined.

Such arrangements may involve the creation of a working party made up of representatives from management, the workforce, unions and occupational health and safety staff, the members of which will collectively review the identified needs, select an appropriate option, define clear, realistic objectives and assess needed resources in both human and financial terms. This sort of collaboration can do much to enhance understanding, to foster agreement and to maintain good industrial relations. A comprehensive approach should enable all sectors of the workforce to become involved and actively to participate in the health-promotion activity.

Implicit within any strategy designed to promote the health of a workforce is the need for a clearly presented plan of the proposed activity.

PLANNING

In order to obtain permission and financial support from senior management, OH practitioners are frequently required to submit a written justification detailing the aim, objectives, methods to be employed, resources required, method of evaluation, timing of the event and an outline of the potential benefits of such a programme. Any written proposal should obviously be:

- well-researched;
- well-presented;

- realistic and feasible;
- costed;
- relevant and appropriate;
- clear and concise.

Questions to consider when compiling such a plan could be:

- Will the proposal aid understanding?
- Does it reflect the needs of both management and the workforce?
- Is it participatory? i.e. does the plan involve everyone?
- Are the resources required clearly identified?
- Has it been adequately costed?
- Are the objectives achievable?
- Are the proposed methods acceptable?
- Are there any ethical implications?
- What will the health-promotion activity achieve?
- How will its success be monitored?

The latter point is of vital importance and the method by which the programme will be evaluated should be determined at the planning stage.

EVALUATION

According to Ewles and Simnett (1992) evaluation is concerned with assessing what has been achieved (outcome evaluation) and how it has been achieved (process evaluation). Williams (1987, p. 81) states that the purpose of evaluation is to 'demonstrate whether an activity has been successful or to what degree it has failed to achieve some stated aims' and to do this a workplace health-promotion activity needs to be monitored so as to identify the value and effectiveness of the activity. Other valuable benefits of evaluation include:

- improvement of methods and materials;
- minimization of waste of scarce resources;
- assessment of the activity's ethical justification;
- justification to management of the need for future programmes or needed changes;
- fostering critical self-appraisal.

Evaluation is not only an integral part of any health-promotion activity but it can be applied at different levels: for example, it may be used to test the effectiveness of a workplace smoking policy or of one-to-one health education with a client who requires counselling concerning their smoking habit or of the effectiveness of a workplace 'Smoking Cessation' group. It is also a key aspect in the management of any workplace health-promotion campaign and Table 6.2 provides a checklist for professionals engaged in this activity.

Table 6.2 Checklist for managing a workplace health-promotion programme

---

MANAGING THE PROGRAMME

---

1 Is there a named person clearly responsible for the overall progress of the programme?
2 Has the programme the visible support of management at all levels?
3 Has adequate, long-term funding been allocated?
4 Is the programme flexible enough to respond to changed circumstances and to cater for the range of needs found in the workforce?
5 Have arrangements been made to monitor the effectiveness of the programme?

ACHIEVING GOOD PARTICIPATION RATES

6 Has the active support of the workforce and their representatives been obtained?
7 Have employees been given the opportunity of participating in the design, implementation and evaluation of the programme?
8 Do some activities take place in the Firm's time?
9 Is it clear that confidentiality will be maintained?
10 Have you tried producing materials with a personal touch to attract new participants?

Source: Rowe, G. (1991) Health Education Authority unpublished material used at a conference for OH nurses at the Institute of Advanced Nursing Education, London.

As can be seen from Table 6.2, a key element in the successful outcome of a workplace health-promotion programme is the ability to achieve participation among members of the workforce. This can only be achieved if the occupational health nurse possesses good communication skills and is well-versed in the basic skills of counselling.

COMMUNICATION AND COUNSELLING

As already indicated, educating for and about health should be both a joint venture between the OH nurse and the worker, and one in which mutual respect, trust, commitment and participation are essential elements. Also, the manner in which notions about health are relayed to the workforce is of paramount importance for successful health promotion. Ewles and Simnett (1992, p. 121) describe 'good communication' as 'clear, unambiguous, two-way, constructive exchanges, without distortion of the message between when it is given and when it is received'. From this it can be assumed that promoting health requires professionals who are skilled in the art of effective communication, although it may be conceded that not all nurses possess such skills (Faulkner and Ward, 1983) and poor communication may have presented a barrier to effective health education/promotion among nurses generally (McCleod Clark, Kendall and Haverty, 1987).

Communication skills fundamental to the business of promoting health at work fall into several distinct categories:

- recognition of values, attitudes and beliefs of both the worker group and the OH nurse;
- respect for the autonomous nature of human beings and encouraging individual workers to make their own decisions;
- respect for the knowledge and experience of the recipients of the health-promotion activity;
- recognition of the sociocultural differences that frequently occur among multicultural occupational groups;
- recognition of factors that may lead to a reduction in the ability to communicate e.g. emotional distress, work stress, mental handicap/illness;
- possession of a good understanding of aspects of non-verbal communication e.g. body posture, eye contact, facial expression;
- possession of a sound knowledge which in turn will increase confidence and credibility;
- recognition that effective listening is an 'active' process and one that will enable the OH nurse to help individual workers to identify their needs.

These categories suggest that for the OH nurse to become involved in educating for and about health they require
- an excellent grasp of issues related to health;
- a good knowledge of the workforce;
- a sound understanding of the organization; and
- a command of communication skills.

In OH practice the majority of clients are healthy, discerning individuals for whom independence and autonomy are fundamental to health and well-being. Thus, promoting health by enabling individuals to make informed decisions and exercise some control over their health would seem to be an appropriate aim for OH practitioners. However, making choices can be an extremely difficult task for some and situations may occur in which the OH nurse is required to engage in the role of counsellor.

Many texts have been written on the art and activity of counselling. It is not within the remit of this chapter to explore the counselling role in any depth but solely to consider the purpose and function of counselling in relation to workplace health promotion.

Counselling is a skilled activity, the purpose of which is to help a person in the identification and exploration of personal needs; set goals and identify options; make decisions and develop a plan of action; and consider and select appropriate coping strategies. In occupational health practice the counselling relationship is one of 'helping' in which the aim is to empower the individual worker to promote their own health. To this end the OH nurse needs to marshall the skills which are specific to counselling such as listening 'actively', responding appropriately, reflecting, paraphrasing, clarifying and summarizing, while at the same time remaining aware of any personal limitations in embracing this role.

If the counselling role requires specific skills, so too does the manner in which health promoters attempt to 'get their message across' – i.e. the skills of teaching and learning.

TEACHING AND LEARNING

In common with counselling, teaching and learning skills abound with volumes written on the subject. It is not intended to attempt reiteration here but simply to highlight specific aspects that may require consideration if successful workplace health promotion is to be achieved.

According to Tones, Tilford and Robinson (1990, p. 224), 'the workplace has its own special needs – not least of which is the adoption of teaching methods appropriate to the adult learner'. The specific needs of adult learners has been explored by writers such as Knowles (1980) and Jarvis and Gibson (1985), both of whom emphasized the importance of recognizing that physiological, psychological and social changes necessarily accompany the ageing process. Such changes will affect the way adults learn; and in order to illustrate this latter point, Knowles (1980) attempted to develop a theoretical perspective specifically concerned with the art and science of adult learning, commonly referred to as androgogy.

The theory of androgogy emphasizes:

- the independence of adult learners acquired during maturation;
- the life experiences of adults which provide a valuable resource for learning;
- the readiness of adults to learn, provided the material is relevant to their life situation;
- the need for adults to be able to apply what they learn.

Although androgogy is not without its critics, the assumptions of the theory are important and worthy of consideration when OH practitioners attempt to assess the learning needs of the workforce.

Opportunities for health education in a working environment are several and include:

- serendipitous:
  i.e. chance, unplanned as when a worker attends the OH department for another reason such as health screening;
- planned:
  i.e. formal, large-scale lecture; informal lecture and discussion; small group activity.

Both approaches require teaching and learning strategies that are congruous with the learning needs of the adult worker.

CONCLUSION

Health promotion, as defined in the Ottawa Charter for Health Promotion (WHO, 1986), is the process of enabling people to take control over and improve their health. If this is to be achieved, then greater opportunities with adequate access to health care for all are required as well as the development of 'an environment conducive to health especially in conditions at work and in the home' (WHO, 1984). Thus the creation of a social and economic environment which seeks to protect health at work appears to be becoming increasingly important and it seems likely that the role and value of OH services in this search will become more prominent as the year 2000 draws nearer. Employers are becoming more proactive in their attitudes toward the provision of a healthy working environment and more amenable to suggestions for the development of workplace health policies. Efforts to achieve the WHO Targets 11 and 25, which pertain specifically to *Health for All 2000* (WHO, 1978) in relation to employment, are likely to gather momentum and these events may result in an expansion of policies designed to protect and promote the health of the workforce.

Official figures suggest that about 2% of all deaths in 15–64-year-olds in Britain are directly attributable to work (Jacobsen, Smith and Whitehead, 1991) which in turn suggests that the work environment poses a serious threat to the health and well-being of the British workforce. According to Addenbrookes Hospital Medical School (cited by Jacobsen *et al.* (1991)) there is evidence to suggest that smokers take approximately twice as much sick leave as non-smokers and that smoking is responsible for the loss of 50 million working days each year. In addition, problem drinking has been estimated to cost industry something in the region of £1714 million per annum (Jacobsen, Smith and Whitehead, 1991).

These figures along suggest that much needs to be done to improve the provision of workplace disease prevention and health promotion. The fact that British workplaces provide access to approximately 28 million adults, who may otherwise be difficult to reach, means that the work environment offers unique opportunities for health education, preventive services and measures to afford the workforce greater health protection as well as the opportunity to achieve a better level of health.

This view is endorsed in the recently published *Health Education Authority Strategy 1993–98* (HEA, 1993). The document, a response to the government White Paper *The Health of the Nation* (DOH, 1992), includes proposals for achieving objectives which specifically address issues related to health at work. For example, the document outlines the HEA's commitment to promote opportunities for workplace health promotion to:

- help achieve the targets as outlined in the White Paper (DOH, 1992);
- participate in the Workplace Task Force (DOH, 1992);
- initiate research into methods of assessing organization and employee needs;
- initiate research into the cost-effectiveness of workplace health-promotion activities.

The authors of the HEA document recognize that the social, organizational and physical environments of the workplace have the potential significantly to influence the health and well-being of the working population.

While there is little doubt that the workplace offers much-needed opportunities for health-promotion initiatives, it is salutary that the Report from the Independent Multidisciplinary Committee (Jacobson, Smith and Whitehead, 1991), set up to investigate the state of the nation's health, states: 'insufficient evidence was available upon which to base a detailed strategy for the promotion of occupational health'. Evidently, there is a general lack both of research studies and of evaluation of workplace health-promotion programmes in the UK at the present time.

When considering the development of formal workplace policies, such as those on smoking, Moreton and East's (1982) research (cited in Jacobson, Smith and Whitehead, 1991) identifies the startling finding: 'a lack of occupational health staff with appropriate communication skills is a major bar to developing such policies'. Admittedly, this was reported some ten years ago but there is no research evidence to suggest that this position has substantially changed.

It is clear, then, that research into workplace health promotion in the UK, although urgently required, is still in its infancy and is sadly lacking. To conduct health-promotion research the researcher needs to gain access to and acceptance from management, the workforce and the unions. Who are better placed to do this than well-prepared occupational health nurses? Knowledge of the organization, of the working population and the work environment, coupled with organizational, communication, counselling, teaching, research, evaluation and policy-making skills, places the occupational health nurse in a unique position to take a leading role in the practice of and research into workplace health promotion.

REFERENCES

Archer, H.M. (1983) A study of the impact of continuing education on occupational health nursing practice. *Occupational Health Nursing*, **31**(2), 15–27.

Ashton, D. (1989) Worksite health promotion – whose responsibility? *Occupational Health Review*, **22**, 26–7.

Bowling, A. (1983) Teamwork in primary health care. *Nursing Times*, **79**(48), 56–9.

Brennan, A.J.J. (1983) Health and fitness boom moves into corporate America. *Occupational Health and Safety*, **54**(7), 38–45.

Crawford, R. (1977) You are a danger to your health: the ideology and politics of victim blaming. *International Journal of Health Services*, **7**(4), 663–80.

Christenson, G.M. and Kiefhaber, A. (1988) The national survey of worksite health promotion activities. *AAOHN Journal*, **36**(6), 262–5.

Department of Health (1992) *The Health of the Nation*, HMSO, London.

Downie, R.S., Fyfe, C. and Tannahill, A. (1990) *Health Promotion: Models and Values*, Oxford University Press, Oxford.

Eriksen, M.P. (1988) Cancer prevention in workplace health promotion. *AAOHN Journal*, **36**(6), 266–70.

Ewles, L. and Simnett, I. (1992) *Promoting Health: A Practical Guide* (2nd edn), Scutari, London.

Faulkner, A. and Ward, L. (1983) Nurses as health educators in relation to smoking. *Nursing Times Occasional Paper*, **79**(8), 47–8.

Fielding, J.E. (1990) Worksite health promotion programs in the United States: progress, lessons and challenges. *Health Promotion International*, **5**(1), 75–84.

Fielding, J.E. and Breslow, L. (1983) Health promotion programs sponsored by California employers. *American Journal of Public Health*, **73**(5), 538–42.

Gordon, J. (1987) Workplace health promotion: the right idea in the wrong place. *Health Education Research*, **2**(1), 69–71.

Gott, M. and O'Brien, M. (1989) *The Role of the Nurse in Health Promotion*, Interim Report, Open University Press, Milton Keynes.

Great Britain, Parliament (1986) *The Social Security Act*, HMSO, London.

Health Education Authority (1993) *Health Education Authority Strategy for 1993–98*, HEA, London.

Hunt, M.W. (1974) *An analysis of factors influencing teamwork in general medical practice*, M.Phil. Thesis, University of Edinburgh.

IRS Employment Trends (1989) Health promotion at work: 1. *IRS Employment Trends*, **438**, 5–11.

IRS Employment Trends (1989) Health promotion at work: 2. *IRS Employment Trends*, **443**, 13–14.

Jacobson, B., Smith, A. and Whitehead, M. (eds) (1991) *The nation's health: a strategy for the 1990s: a report from an independent multidisciplinary committee*, (revised edn), King Edward's Hospital Fund, London.

Jarvis, P. and Gibson, S. (1985) *The Teacher Practitioner in Nursing, Midwifery and Health Visiting*, Croom Helm, London.

Knowles, M. (1980) *The modern practice of adult education* (2nd edn), Association Press, Chicago.

Legge, R. (1934) *Industrial Maladies*, Oxford University Press, London.

McCleod Clark, J., Kendall, S. and Haverty, S. (1987) Helping nurses develop their health education role: a framework for training. *Nurse Education Today*, **7**(2), 63–8.

Molle, C.D. and Allan, J. (1989) The need for a more holistic health care system. *AAOHN Journal*, **37**(12), 518–25.

Molloy, J. (1990) *'Giving health to the workforce': A study to determine the extent to which the health education component of the occupational health nursing course meets the needs of practising occupational health nurses*, MSc Thesis, University of London.

Morris, L.I. (1985) A conceptual model for occupational health nursing practice. *Occupational Health Nursing*, **33**(2), 66–70.

Popp, R.A. (1989) An overview of occupational health promotion. *AAOHN Journal*, **37**(4), 113–20.

Radford, J. (ed.) (1990) *Recent Advances in Nursing: Occupational Health Nursing*, Churchill Livingstone, Edinburgh.

Ross, F. (1987) *Evaluation of a Drug Guide in Primary Care*, PhD. Thesis, University of London.

Rowe, G. (1991) Health Education Authority unpublished material used at a conference for OH nurses at The Institute of Advanced Nursing Education, RCN, London.

Schenck, A.P., Thomas, R.P., Holhbaum, G.M. and Beliczri, L.S. (1987) A labor and industry focus on education: using baseline survey data in program design. *Health Education Research*, **2**(1), 33–44.

Schilling, R.S.F. (1989) Health protection and promotion at work. *British Journal of Industrial Medicine*, **46**(10), 683–8.

Seedhouse, D. (1986) Health: a universal concern. *Nursing Times*, **82**(4), 36–8.

Selleck, C.S., Sirles, A.T. and Newman, K.D. (1989) Health promotion at the workplace. *AAOHN Journal*, **37**(10), 412–22.

Shephard, R.J. (1986) *Fitness and Health in Industry*, Karger, New York.

Smogor, J. and Macrina, D.M. (1987) Problems in worksite health promotion: the perspective of small business. *AAOHN Journal*, **35**(5), 224–8.

Tannahill, A. (1985) What is health promotion? *Health Education Journal*, **44**(4), 167–8.

Taylor, J.R. (1987) Health promotion in a single-nurse unit. *AAOHN Journal*, **35**(5), 229–32.

Tones, K., Tilford, S. and Robinson, Y. (1990) *Health Education: Effectiveness and Efficiency*, Chapman & Hall, London.

US Department of Health, Education and Welfare (1979) *Healthy People: The Surgeon General's Report on Health Promotion and Disease Prevention*, Washington DC.

Watterson, A. (1986) Occupational health and illness: the politics of hazard education, in *The Politics of Health Education: Raising the Issues* (eds Rodmell, S. and Watt, A.) Routledge and Kegan Paul, London, pp. 76–99.

Webb, T. *et al.* (1988) *Health at Work: A Report on Health Promotion in the Workplace* (Research Report 22) Health Education Authority, London.

Williams, T. (1987) Health education in secondary schools, in *Health Education in Schools*, 2nd edn (eds David, K. and Williams, T.), Harper and Row, London, pp. 60–85.

World Health Organisation (1978) *Primary Health Care: Report of the International Conference on Primary Health Care, Alma Ata, USSR 6–12 September 1978*, WHO, Geneva.

World Health Organisation (1984) Health promotion: a WHO discussion document on the concept and principles. *Journal of the Institute of Health Education*, **23**(1), 431–5.

World Health Organisation (1986) *The Ottawa Charter for Health Promotion*, Copenhagen, WHO.

7

Employment law

Michael Whincup

INTRODUCTION

Every day in British industry an average of four people die of injuries or industrial diseases. In the course of a year, tens of thousands are injured. Some 23 million working days are lost, ten or more times the number currently lost by strike action.[1] What can the law do to stop or reduce this mayhem? One might at first be tempted to say 'very little', if only because the figures have not greatly altered despite the wave of legislation which followed the 'new deal' of the Health and Safety at Work Act in 1974. But common sense tells us that if it were not for the law, things would be very much worse. In fact, it is really only the pressure of the law which in the long run can change our attitudes and actions. It is very important therefore to understand how the law works, and what might be done to strengthen and improve it.

CIVIL AND CRIMINAL LAW

Essentially the law works in two different ways, seeking so far as practicable to prevent accidents happening in the first place, and to compensate the victims as and when they do. The preventive approach is that of the criminal law; the compensatory, that of civil law. Breaches of the Factories Act 1961, Offices, Shops and Railway Premises Act 1963, Mines and Quarries Act 1954 and similar legislation – but not, as we shall see, the Health and Safety at Work Act of 1974 – have both civil and criminal consequences.

Each method has its own advantages and disadvantages in

terms of accident prevention. The great merit of the criminal law is, of course, that the Health and Safety inspectors do not need to wait for accidents to happen, but can take or threaten action as soon as they see unsafe places of work or unsafe working practices. The problem is that the inspectors are relatively few in number – some 600 or 700 – and can visit each place of work for which they are responsible only around once every four years. They have neither the time nor the resources to follow up and prosecute every breach of the law they find. And when they do prosecute, they have often been disappointed by the trivial fines imposed by magistrates on the guilty parties.

THE COMMON LAW

In practice, it is the civil law, whose purpose is not to punish the wrongdoer but to compensate the victim, which is much the more often invoked. Rights to compensation are given not only by the Acts of Parliament we have mentioned, but also by the common law – those principles of law developed independently of Parliament by the judges. Insurance against such claims, which is required by law,[2] is a substantial burden on employers, and in turn an incentive for them to take safety precautions.

The main disadvantages of civil claims are that it may be many years before they come to trial and the hazards in question can be examined, and, for reasons discussed below, many claims fail and people most in need may get nothing. Without legal aid or trade-union assistance, the costs may be ruinous. The confrontational nature of these cases also means that each side keeps its information secret from the other until the day of the trial. There is then no common interest in finding out how the accident happened and trying to ensure that it does not happen again. And since the object of the claim is to get as much money as possible for one's injuries, the injured party has no incentive to get better. On the contrary, he or she has every reason to rub salt into the wound in order to be at his or her worst on that day. These consequences are perverse, to say the least. We should also mention in passing that rights to compensation are quite separate and distinct from rights to remain in employment. Employers are entitled to dismiss employees who are unable to do their work, whatever the cause of their disability.[3]

For the moment, however, we must consider the system as it

is, and not as we might like it to be. The next step, therefore, is to distinguish between the obligations imposed by Act of Parliament and those imposed by the common law. Until quite recently, a feature of our safety legislation has been in its very limited and detailed effect. Rules were devised by Parliament from time to time to meet specific problems arising out of particular types of work, at the expense of more general or overriding safety duties. That situation has now been changed by the Health and Safety at Work Act and the regulations made under it. The common law, on the other hand, has always laid down very general principles of liability, applicable to any and every kind of employment. In a brief account of the law such as this we cannot do more than indicate the range of liabilities covered by statute, noting the most important of the new regulations passed in accordance with European Community Directives, but we can usefully try to explain the all-embracing rules of common law.

Reasonable care

There are in fact two such basic rules. The first is that **employers must take reasonable care for the safety of their employees**: no more; no less. This fundamental and deceptively simple principle was introduced by the judges over 150 years ago. Breach of the rule gives rise to a claim for damages by the injured worker, to compensate for pain and suffering and loss of employment. The novelty and the importance of the Health and Safety at Work Act was that it made this same civil duty enforcable also by the criminal law, thus greatly extending the inspectorate's previously limited preventive powers. Section 2 of the Act requires employers to ensure 'so far as is reasonably practicable' the safety, health and welfare of their employees. Because this is essentially the same duty as that already imposed by the common law, it was not necessary for the Act to give further rights to compensation to workers injured by breaches of the Act.

For the purposes of both civil and criminal law, therefore, we must try to define what is meant by reasonable care. We might note first that this is not a rule peculiar to employment. It applies in all relationships where there is a risk of injury. Road users must take reasonable care to avoid injuring other road users; manufacturers must take reasonable care for the safety of users of their products; doctors and nurses must take reasonable care of their patients, and so on. In all cases the effect of the rule is that one must, so to say, 'do one's best' to avoid injuring others. Even so, accidents may still happen. Clearly there can be no guarantee of safety, at work or elsewhere. If the injured party cannot prove the other side at fault, he or she has no claim for compensation.

What then must the injured party prove in order to establish negligence? The mere fact of accident or injury is not sufficient. It must be shown that the defendant employer (or driver, doctor, etc.) failed to do what a reasonable person would have done in the circumstances, or did what a reasonable person would not have done. This depends very much upon the judge's assessment of the facts of the particular case. The factors that influence his/ her decision are largely matters of common sense. They include, for example, the likelihood or otherwise of the accident (on the basis that a reasonable man or woman would do more to avoid a likely accident than an unlikely one), its potential seriousness, the obviousness of the risk, the cost of taking precautions and the inherent risk of the activity in question. The judge must weigh these factors one against the other. His/her decision is often quite unpredictable.

It might be helpful to say a little more here about two of these factors: the obviousness or otherwise of the danger, and the inherent risk aspect. A danger which is immediately obvious to an employer, and which he/she must therefore do his/her best to reduce or remove, is probably equally obvious to the employee. That employee must then take appropriate pre-cautions for his/her own safety. If he/she ignores or forgets the danger he/she may be held wholly or partly to blame for the resulting accident. He/she may be said to have agreed to run the risk – though that requires more than mere knowledge of its existence – and in that case will have no claim at all. If he/ she has simply been careless, his/her contributory negligence will cost him/her whatever proportion of his/her damages the judge thinks represents his/her share of the blame. This may range anywhere between 5% or 10% and 100%. On principle such deductions may appear quite reasonable, but they are essentially arbitrary and can have disproportionately disastrous conse-quences for employees. In a dangerous situation created by many years of managerial indifference, for example, an employee might suffer severe injury because of a moment's miscalculation or oversight. A judge might then hold him/her, say, 50% to blame, and so reduce his/her award from £100,000 to £50,000. Decisions of this kind, which seem to take no real account of the employer's blameworthiness, and are in effect swingeing fines upon the employee and his/her family, are by no means uncommon.

As regards inherent risk, the point is simply that every activity involves a degree of danger which is irreducible. Anyone whose job it is to lift or carry goods, for example, runs a risk of strain or dislocation even though the goods themselves are not heavy or unmanagable. Anyone who uses a hammer and chisel or who knocks a nail into a piece of wood runs the risk of injuring himself or herself severely. If such injury occurs it is very unlikely that anyone else can be blamed, and so there is no redress for the injury, however serious it might be.

With these considerations in mind, let us look at some specific problem areas and the decided cases that illustrate the general rule. For the sake of convenience we can divide the cases under the headings of safety of premises, plant, fellow employees and system of work.

Safe premises

Employers must take reasonable care to ensure the place of work is safe. This obligation requires a careful assessment of risks arising from the structure of the place, its layout and the processes carried on within it, and appropriate preventive action. Typical problems concern the maintenance of passageways and stairs. If an employee slips on a pool of oil or water on a factory floor, is the employer necessarily liable? The gangway is supposed to be safe, but, as we said above, the fact of an accident there does not prove the employer has been negligent in failing to maintain it properly. The outcome of a claim of this kind would depend on such factors as the length of time the oil or water had been on the floor, how it came to be there, whether anyone knew or should have known it was there, and what if any opportunity there had been to clean it up. If, for instance, a passing fork-lift truck had leaked a little oil on to the floor immediately after it had been cleaned, and an employee following the truck had slipped on the oil, it would hardly be possible to blame the employer. To hold him/her liable would in effect require him/her to catch every drop of oil or water before it hit the floor, which is clearly impossible. Reasonable care requires the employer only to do that which is practicable in the circumstances. The standard is essentially a compromise between what is desirable and what is feasible on the facts of each case.

The basic common-law duty is reinforced by specific statutory provision, enforceable also by criminal sanctions. In particular, the Workplace (Health, Safety and Welfare) Regulations 1992 require that floors, steps, passages and gangways be soundly constructed, properly maintained and as far as reasonably practicable kept free from obstructions and slippery substances. They require safe ways into and out of the workplace, and separation of vehicle and pedestrian routes, again so far as is reasonably practicable. The regulations also make more general provision for standards of lighting, cleanliness, temperature, work space, and eating, washing and toilet facilities, etc. These and several other of the new regulations we shall mention are accompanied by approved codes of practice which explain how they are to be fulfilled.

There have been countless common-law cases on these issues over the years. *Latimer v. A.E.C.*, 1953,[4] is a leading case on the balancing of the various elements of liability. Here a factory floor was flooded after a storm. The employer had two courses of action open to him: either to close the factory altogether, or to try to make the floor safe by putting down all the available sawdust. He decided to stay open and to put down sawdust. Unfortunately there was not quite enough to go around, and an employee slipped and injured himself on an untreated part of the floor. The judge rejected the employee's claim. He said it would have been disproportionately expensive to close the factory in order to avoid a slight risk of a slight injury.

A more straightforward example is *Bell v. Department of Health and Social Security*, 1989.[5] The area round a much-used office tea machine on a marble-type floor was often slippery. The employer knew of the danger and put up a notice urging employees to take care. No other precautions were taken. The employer was held liable for the ensuing accident. A warning notice is not by itself a sufficient precaution against a continuing and remediable danger.

The employer's duty extends to the provision of safe ways into and out of the place of work, but again only so far as is reasonable. In *Martin v. Greater Glasgow Health Board*, 1977,[6] a student nurse fell over the bannisters in a nurses' home. She lost her claim because she could not show the bannisters were significantly lower than in other such institutions, and in any case thousands of people had used the stairway in the past without mishap. Falls on snow or ice on company car parks, etc., have led to many claims – whose results are again difficult if not impossible to predict. In *Gitsham v. Pearce*, 1992,[7] the employer's efforts to keep pathways on an open site safe were nullified by the severe weather. He escaped liability accordingly.

Responsibility for the safety of the workplace is not confined to the employer's own immediate premises, but covers anywhere he/she sends his employees to work. In *Hawes v. Railway Executive*, 1952,[8] the plaintiff was a ganger, doing minor running repairs on a stretch of electrified railway line. He slipped or tripped and was electrocuted. His widow claimed damages for her loss. She could prove the likelihood of such an accident, its seriousness, the defendants' knowledge of the risk, and also that the risk could have been eliminated if the employers had turned the current off. All these points are, as we have seen, the ingredients of a successful claim. But her claim failed, because of the one remaining issue – the cost of turning off the current. If it were turned off at all, it would have to be off for everyone working at any time on or near the track, which would have meant total dislocation of the service. The court held that this 'social cost', as we may call it, was too high a price. *Hawes* illustrates that society's demands make many accidents more or less inevitable, and at the same time shows that those who are injured or the dependents of those who are killed in such accidents will get no compensation whatever.

When an employer sends his/her men to work on someone else's premises, e.g., to do building or repair work there, he/she is still responsible for their safety. In practice his/her responsibility is much reduced by the obvious limits on his/her ability to remedy structural defects or control unsafe working practices. If his/her employees are to work on the site for any length of time he/she might have to visit it beforehand to see whether there are any unusual dangers, but that could not be necessary before visits to private houses by, say, window cleaners or social workers. If precautions are needed they might take the form of safety equipment, as in *General Cleaning Contractors v. Christmas*,

1953,[9] or advice or instructions to the occupier. The occupier might share in the liability for the accident as in *Smith v. Austin Lifts*, 1959,[10] where he failed to act on the employer's warning of a dangerous lift on the premises, or he might be wholly liable, or, of course, as we have emphasized, the facts may be such that neither employer nor occupier is to blame.

The difficulties of deciding on liability in these cases where employees work away from their base are shown in *McDermid v. Nash*, 1987,[11] and *Cook v. Square D*, 1992.[12] In *McDermid* the plaintiff was sent to work as a deckhand on a tug owned by another company. He was under the control of the captain, himself an employee of the other company. The plaintiff was injured because of an unsafe system of work adopted by the captain. The House of Lords held the defendants liable, on the ground that their responsibility for their employees' safety was a personal one and could not be delegated to someone else to fulfil (a decision followed by the Court of Appeal in *Morris v. Breaveglen*, 1992).[13] In *Cook* the plaintiff was an engineer, sent to work in Saudi Arabia. He was injured by falling into a hole in the floor of the room where he worked. He knew the hole was there, to give access to cables underneath. Undeniably the hole made the floor unsafe, but the employers nonetheless escaped liability. The Court of Appeal said they had taken care in ensuring the site occupiers were responsible contractors, and could not reasonably be held to blame for day-to-day hazards on this distant site. This seems to be the right decision, but is not easy to reconcile with *McDermid*. If and in so far as the defendants in that case satisfied themselves of the captain's competence – and they had no reason to doubt it – what more could they reasonably have been expected to do to safeguard their employee?

Safe plant and equipment

This sub-heading covers every kind of equipment used by employees in the course of their work; not only production machinery but also, for example, ladders, seats, protective clothing, works transport – and even, in *Knowles v. Liverpool City Council*, 1992,[14] a flagstone.

Common-law liabilities in this area are supplemented by numerous criminally enforceable statutory provisions, both general and particular in their scope. For present purposes the most far-reaching are the Provision and Use of Work Equipment Regulations 1992. The regulations define 'work equipment' as any machinery, appliance, apparatus, tool or assembly of components functioning as a whole. The equipment must be constructed, adapted and maintained so as to be suitable for its purposes and used only for those purposes. Suitable information and instruction must be given to users. More detailed rules affect the construction and use of dangerous machinery, repealing the complex provisions of the Factories Act. We refer below to other recent regulations on manual handling, protective clothing and display screens, and bear in mind that many other products and processes are similarly regulated.

As with premises, so a process or item of equipment is not unsafe merely because it causes injury, but only if the employer knows or ought to know it is potentially harmful and there is some precaution he/she can reasonably be expected to take to reduce the risk. Recent instances include liability for unsuitable seating causing repetitive strain injury – *McSherry v. British Telecom*, 1992,[15] – and for failing to provide ear protectors for shipyard workers after the danger of deafness in this kind of work had been generally recognized: *Baxter v. Harland and Wolff*, 1990.[16] In *Pape v. Cumbria County Council*, 1991,[17] cleaners were given gloves, but not told to wear them nor instructed in the dangers of chemical cleaners. Again the employers were liable.

The key question in all these cases is, as we have said, whether or when the employer knew or ought to have known of the hazard. Risks which are not immediately obvious may come to light, for example, through employees' complaints. We note here that complaints do not of themselves prove equipment is unsafe. Clearly an employer fails to investigate a complaint at his/her peril, but on investigation he/she might find the complaint unjustified, or the proposed precaution excessive (e.g., provision of safety boots where there is only a very small risk of slight injury, or of barrier cream for every dirty job involving some slight risk of dermatitis: *Darvill v. Hampton*, 1972).[18] In that case he/she need not take any further action and so he/she would not be liable even if by some mischance an injury did subsequently occur in exactly the circumstances complained of. Another possibility is that an employer might decide to modify or replace certain items of equipment. If he/she does so, that does not prove that those items were dangerous. Otherwise, of course, he/she would have no incentive to update and improve his/her plant; indeed, he/she would have every reason not to.

Employers must keep up to date with health and safety developments in their industries. This duty affects not only changes in the law such as the 1992 Display Screen Equipment Regulations, which lay down detailed rules as to the suitability of equipment and workstations and the comfort of operators), but also obliges them to read and follow the relevant codes and advisory materials published by the Health and Safety Executive, trade journals and the like. The availability of such information has been most important in enabling judges to decide the earliest dates at which employers should have taken precautions against risks such as deafness or vibration white finger in their particular industries: *Baxter,* above; *Bowman v. Harland & Wolff,* 1992.[19] On the other hand, employers could not reasonably be expected either to know or, still less, to act immediately on the results of research published only in medical journals – unless, perhaps, they employ occupational health practitioners: *Wright v. Dunlop,* 1972.[20]

We note finally the rule applicable where injury is caused by a hidden defect in equipment supplied by a third party, a manufacturer. If the danger is completely hidden from and unknowable by the employer, he/she could not be liable at common law for an injury. In theory the injured employee would have to discover the identity of the manufacturer and sue him/her instead. In practice it might be very difficult for him/her to do so and in any case his/her claim might be barred by the passage of time. To overcome these problems, the Employers' Liability (Defective Equipment) Act 1969 makes the employer strictly liable in this situation, and leaves him/her to seek what redress he/she can from the manufacturer, e.g., in a breach of contract action.

Safe fellow-employees

Many injuries are caused by untrained or inadequately supervised employees. Employees must be qualified for the work they do, or work under instruction. Training his/her employees in safe working practices is clearly a vital part of an employer's responsibilities at common law. The duty is endorsed by the criminal law in s.2 of the Health and Safety at Work Act, and more specifically by regulation 11 of the Management of Health and Safety at Work Regulations 1992, described below. It is particularly important to ensure the competence of employees in charge of safety and training. In *Birnie v. Ford*, 1960,[21] the employer was held liable for injuries that could have been prevented by a more competent safety officer.

An employee may still be a danger to others despite his training if he/she has some kind of personality defect; if he/she is, for example, was quick tempered or aggressive, a bully or a practical joker. When through previous incidents and complaints an employer learns that he/she has such an employee, he/she must take appropriate precautions. Sometimes a warning might be sufficient; more probably dismissal will be the only realistic solution: *Hudson v. Ridge*, 1957.[22] An employer would be liable if he/she knew his/her workers forced new entrants to go through dangerous 'initiation' rituals, but made no attempt to stop them. Problems of stress caused by conflicts of personality, or by pressures of work generally, are obviously more difficult to resolve. But on principle an employer could be liable for an employee's nervous collapse if he/she made no attempt to deal with a potentially injurious situation of which he/she knew or should have known.

Another possible cause of danger would arise where an employee is suffering from an illness, or drink or drug addiction. Generally speaking, illness or addiction must be treated more carefully and considerately than misconduct, perhaps allowing for medical care and counselling, but still not to the point of seriously endangering other people. An important point arises here in connection with employees who are or are believed to be HIV positive or AIDS sufferers. Other employees may feel themselves at risk and refuse to work with a sufferer. The Department of Employment's guide, *AIDS and Employment*, says it is the employer's responsibility to educate his/her workforce to understand that the risk of infection in most occupations is almost non-existent, and that if he/she fails to do this he/she may well be acting unfairly if he/she dismisses a suspect or sufferer because of pressure from other employees.

Safe systems of work

This is the last but in many respects the most extensive aspect of the employer's overall duty of care. It concerns his/her responsibility to 'set the stage' for safety; to ensure that work is properly organized and supervised, and in particular that safety equipment is provided and used wherever necessary.

The requirements have recently been set down in detail in the Management of Health and Safety at Work Regulations 1992, enforceable only by prosecution by the Health and Safety Executive. Excluding work on seagoing ships, the regulations oblige employers to make a 'suitable and sufficient' assessment of the risks to which his/her employees and any contractors or other third parties are exposed by his/her operations in order to decide on the appropriate safety precautions. Self-employed workers must do the same for their own benefit. Where there are five or more employees, the main findings of the assessment must be stated in writing, specifying any group of workers especially at risk, together with the arrangements made for preventive and protective measures.

In particular, these measures include 'appropriate health surveillance' – the first general recognition in English law of the importance of occupational health practitioners – and the appointment of a sufficient number of 'competent persons' (such as safety officers) to help the employer to meet his obligations. Procedures for serious and imminent dangers and for danger areas must be established, enabling employees and others to stop work if need be. Employers must provide employees with 'comprehensive and relevant' information on the risks identified and the precautions to be taken against them. Co-operation and co-ordination is required between two or more employers sharing a work place. All necessary safety information must be given to contractors and their employees working on the site. General health and safety training duties are imposed, to be fulfilled during working hours. Employees must use the safety equipment provided, and report new hazards and any shortcomings in existing safety arrangements.

It will be seen that many of the issues identified by these regulations are very much those affecting first- or middle-line managers, requiring from them in particular decisions as to which employees need instruction and supervision, the appropriate precautions and the level of supervision suitable in each case – decisions which may differ from day to day or job to job. New employees generally need more attention than those with many years' experience, but on the other hand familiarity with a job may lessen even the most experienced employee's awareness of danger. Against that again, management should be able to rely at least to some extent on employees exercising their own common sense to protect themselves. We bear in mind the judge's memorable remarks in *Boyle v. Kodak*, 1967,[23] on the question whether the plaintiff and his mate should have been told to go up some steps in order to lash the top of a ladder: 'That sort of thing is a thing which employers cannot decently and properly say to a man of intelligence and experience . . . They would be quite rightly annoyed to have a foreman standing over them nursing them to see whether they were doing the job properly. Quite rightly they could tell him to go away and have a cup of tea.'

There are many illustrations of the problems posed by these conflicting interests. We note first some examples of unsuccessful claims. Employers have escaped liability for failing to tell employees not to put their weight on obviously rotten wood, or not to pour naptha on to a fire, or to stop work if overcome by heat, or how to get on a works bus, or how to avoid a rush into the canteen. In *Brennan v. Techno*, 1962,[24] a skilled steel erector was told to fix a block and tackle on a roof truss 14ft. above ground. He climbed out along the truss instead of using a ladder, and fell. No blame was attached to his employer for not telling him to use a ladder, or suggesting that a ladder might be safer. In *Langan v. French*, 1961,[25] a labourer instructed to cut a pipe with a hacksaw used a hammer instead, and so suffered injury from steam in the pipe which he would not otherwise have suffered. His employer was held under no duty to tell him of the danger of using a hammer, since otherwise every employer could be liable for failing to warn every employee against each and every danger that might arise if even the simplest and clearest instructions were disobeyed or carried out in some entirely different way. When an employee was sent to work in another country where car insurance was not compulsory, the employer was not liable for failing to warn him against driving uninsured, or for not taking out a policy for him: *Reid v. Rush and Tompkins*, 1990.[26]

A great many cases arise from back injuries, which result every day in some 80,000 absences from work. Liability for these sprains and strains and dislocations may be very difficult to determine. A claim might well be rejected if the load itself was not unusually heavy, and the real cause of the injury was an awkward movement or the poor posture of the employee – the inherent risk problem mentioned earlier. In an Australian case the judge rejected the claim on these grounds:

> Reduced to its simple essentials, the employer is said to have been negligent in requiring the plaintiff, who was employed as labourer, and a fellow employee to lift a sheet of metal weighing 160 pounds. Stated baldly thus, the proposition is a startling one. To assert that a labourer may recover damages because he is required to perform labour of a moderate kind is completely insupportable. It is little short of ludicrous.

One occupation in particular which is constantly troubled by risks of back injury is that of nursing. It is unrealistic to suppose that employers could provide hoists or other aids every time patients have to be moved or lifted – but equally clear that help of some sort should be readily available whenever a nurse reasonably fears that they might not be able to manage. The difficulties were illustrated in *Steenhuis v. S.E. Metropolitan Regional Health Authority*, 1975.[27] A nurse here injured her back while helping another nurse to lift an 18-stone patient. The injury ended her nursing career and left her in constant pain. She claimed that a hoist should have been provided for such a heavy patient. But she had not been lifting the patient by herself and an employer might well have assumed that two experienced nurses could handle a weight of this kind. Rejecting her claim, the judge said it was not reasonable to expect hospital authorities to provide a hoist 'just because there was a risk that a nurse might injure her back when lifting a patient'.

Apart from the inherent risk aspect, lifting-injury cases usually fall into one of two categories. In the first, the evidence will suggest that the employee should have seen for themselves that the load was too heavy to be moved or lifted single-handed. The onus would then be on the employee to refuse to do the job without help. If they went ahead without help, the employer would not be liable. In the second category of cases we find the employee working under pressure or having no choice but to get on with the job and run the risk of injury. On those facts the claim should succeed, in whole or part.

In *Osarak v. Hawker Siddeley*, 1982,[28] for instance, a tea lady was awarded damages for tennis elbow caused by constant lifting of a 6-pint teapot. The employer had ignored her complaints, though supported by medical evidence. Equally convincing is *Goodfellow v. Essex County Council*, 1980,[29] where a cleaner at a fire station won her claim for injuries sustained when she hauled her 89-pound equipment up two flights of stairs. Her employer had not ensured that help was available when it was obviously needed. She had in fact asked the firemen for assistance, but they were having a tea break at the time and explained to her that it was against union rules to help her.

This whole area of risk has been reconsidered and the law strengthened to some extent by more new rules, the Manual Handling Operations Regulations, 1992, enforceable both civilly and criminally. The regulations, which replace long-standing provisions of the Factories Act, say that employers must so far as is reasonably practicable try to avoid the need for employees to undertake manual handling operations at work which may injure them. If such operations cannot be avoided, then the risks must be assessed according to the nature of the task, the load, the environment and individual capability – elements detailed in the regulations. The risks thus established must be reduced to and maintained at the lowest reasonably practicable level. Employees must follow the systems of work laid down. The self-employed have the same responsibilities to themselves as are imposed on employers.

The importance of training in safe lifting and handling techniques has often been emphasized. A recent example is *Ping v. Esselte-Letraset*, 1992.[30] Employees in this case were exposed by their work to risks of tenosynovitis and similar upper-limb disorders, which eventually developed. The employer was held to blame for not warning them of the risks before they began work, explaining the need to report any pain immediately and seek medical advice, and for not providing regular reminders.

One of the most important and difficult aspects of the employer's duty concerns the provision of safety clothing – goggles, gloves, hard hats, boots, etc. – and the level of supervision necessary to see that this equipment is used. Many injuries arise through employees' failure to take the necessary precautions.

How far is the employer supposed to go to ensure his/her orders are obeyed?

The common-law duty to provide such equipment, supplemented by regulations for various trades, has been reinforced by the Personal Protective Equipment at Work Regulations, 1992. The regulations require employers to provide 'suitable personal protective equipment' where work cannot otherwise be made safe. Self-employed people must provide and use such equipment for themselves. Suitability depends on the nature of the risk, ergonomic requirements, the relevant employee's state of health, correct fitting and the practicability of preventing or controlling the risk. The very specific and individual nature of the duty is shown by the case of *Paris v. Stepney Borough Council*, 1951,[31] where an employer was held liable for not providing goggles for a one-eyed employee, though the danger was so small that he would not have needed to supply them for a normally sighted employee.

The regulations further require employers and the self-employed to assess the suitability and compatibility of the equipment with any other necessary safety equipment before choosing it. The equipment must be maintained and replaced as necessary and kept in appropriate accommodation when not in use. Employees must be adequately instructed in the use of the equipment and as to the risks it is intended to avoid, and must report any defects in it. Regulation 10 then seeks to answer the crucial question of compulsion by saying: 'Every employer shall take all reasonable steps to ensure that any personal protective equipment ... is properly used.' And correspondingly: 'Every employee shall use any [such] equipment' in accordance with his training and instructions.

It will be seen that this statutory duty to take 'all reasonable steps' is basically the same as that of the common law, and leaves us little the wiser as to what should or must be done to ensure compliance. But guidance has been provided by a number of leading cases, including *Woods v. Durable Suites*, 1953.[32] The plaintiff here was an experienced glue-spreader in the defendant's furniture factory. He had been fully and personally instructed in the dangers of dermatitis and told to use the barrier cream and washing facilities provided. A poster campaign reinforced the message. Unknown to his supervisors he did not use the barrier cream or washing facilities as often as he should have done, and contracted dermatitis. He sued his employers for failing to provide a level of supervision sufficient to ensure that he took the necessary precautions. Not surprisingly, his claim was rejected. The judge said: 'There is no duty at common law to stand over workmen of age and experience.'

In contrast is *Crookall v. Vickers Armstrong*, 1955,[33] where the employer was liable for making only a 'half-hearted' attempt to get his employees to wear respirators against the danger of silicosis. It was the employer's duty, said the judge, to 'encourage and exhort' his employees with 'earnestness and ardour' to take the necessary precautions. Periodic inspections and ineffectual warnings were not sufficient.

The plaintiff in *Qualcast v. Haynes*, 1959,[34] was a foundry worker who was injured by a spillage of molten metal. He was not wearing the safety boots which he knew were available. The court held that employers who provided the appropriate equipment were not then obliged to try to force experienced employees to use it in order to protect themselves against obvious hazards. To hold otherwise, as the House of Lords said in another such case, would be to reduce the employment relationship to that of 'nursemaid and imbecile child'.

In *Berry v. Stone Manganese Marine*, 1971,[35] one of the first major cases on industrial deafness, the employer was again held to blame for failure both to issue ear protectors at the right time and to take any active interest in seeing they were worn. A similar decision was given in *Baxter v. Harland and Wolff*, 1990.[36] (The general problem of industrial deafness has been recognized only relatively recently. Specific duties to assess the danger, reduce sound levels and provide ear protectors are now imposed by the Noise at Work Regulations 1989.)

These cases may seem difficult to reconcile, but we can in fact draw four useful guidelines from them. The first is that employers must ensure their employees know the dangers of their work. If the dangers are hidden – as with dermatitis, silicosis and deafness – employers must run all-out safety campaigns to try to ensure understanding. But if the danger is glaringly obvious, as with molten metal, that kind of campaign is not necessary. Second, employers must ensure their employees know the precautions needed to meet those dangers. Again, if the dangers are hidden, so too may be the need for precautions. The all-out safety campaign should therefore also emphasize the use of safety equipment, combining as appropriate personal instruction, incentive and penalities. Third the precautions must be available. Boots, masks, etc., must be immediately available and if need be, given into the hands of each employee individually. Fourth the employer must in any event ensure that employees know that the precautions are available.

We might be tempted then to propose a fifth rule: that employers must ensure the precautions are actually **used**. But such a rule would be unrealistic. Employers cannot physically force employees to take precautions they do not wish to take. A disobedient employee may be taken off a job, or, ultimately, dismissed, but that of itself does not ensure that they or others take the necessary precautions. It is suggested, therefore, that the four rules above tell us the practical meaning of and limitations on the duty to take reasonable care.

Vicarious liability

The second of the two basic rules of employers' liability is the common-law principle of vicarious liability. This expression means 'liability for another person's wrongdoing'. The rule is that **an employer is liable to anyone injured by the wrongful acts of his employees, committed in the course of their employment**.

Unlike our first rule, which, as we have seen, depends on proof of the employer's negligence, this present principle makes him liable even though he/she is in no way to blame – except perhaps in the sense that since he/she is in overall control of the enterprise he/she must take responsibility if things go wrong. The question is no longer whether the employer has been negligent, but whether his/her employee has. If he/she has, then the employer must compensate the injured party. So in *Lindsay v. Connell*, 1951,[37] the employer was liable where a workman hammering a piece of steel held by another employee negligently hit the other on his finger. Similarly, a pedestrian run down in the street by a careless bus driver would sue the bus company rather than the driver.

From the employer's point of view the rule may well seem harsh and unreasonable, particularly since there is usually little or nothing he could do to prevent these accidents and injuries occurring. But the purpose of the rule is to give the injured party a realistic right to redress. If his or her claim was against the wrongdoer alone it would probably be worthless, since most employees would not have the money to pay large awards of damages. To help the injured party, therefore, the law provides an alternative right of recourse against the employer, who must be insured against such claims (though it should be understood that the fact he is insured does not in any way determine the question whether he is liable). The rule does not, of course, relieve the wrongdoer of liability. The employer may still try to recover from him/her the sum he/she has had to pay to the injured party, and/or he/she might properly dismiss him/her for doing his/her job so badly as to cause injury.

The employer's personal and vicarious liabilities may sometimes overlap. He/she may be personally to blame for an accident at work caused by his/her failure to institute a safe system of supervision, or vicariously liable for the supervisor's failure to do his/her job properly. From the injured worker's point of view the effect is the same. But that is not always the case, and it may be very important to establish which rule is relied on. We mentioned earlier, for example, problems of violence at work. An employer would probably not be vicariously liable for one employee's assault on another, since it would be most unlikely to occur in the course of the wrongdoer's employment, but he/she might be personally liable if, because of previous incidents, he/she knew or should have known this employee was a menace and so should have got rid of him/her.

We see then that the plaintiff in a vicarious liability claim has to prove two basic points. He/she must establish first that the employee committed what we have called a wrongful act, and second, that the act was committed in the course of his/her employment. We consider these requirements now in a little more detail.

By a 'wrongful act' we mean any civil or criminal wrong. Usually the problem arises because of an injury caused by the civil wrong of negligence, but it might equally be a dispute over financial loss caused by a breach of contract or a fraud of some kind. So far as physical injuries are concerned, it is important to remember that they may occur without negligence. In *Lindsay,* above, for example, the employer would not have been liable if the employee could have proved he was using the hammer with every possible care. And if the bus driver mentioned earlier had caused the accident through having a heart attack, it is very unlikely that any claim could be made against the bus company because it is not negligent to have a heart attack.

This question of negligence on the one hand and misadventure or accident on the other is particularly clear, and particularly important, in the medical context. Doctors and nurses are not negligent merely because something goes wrong in the course of treatment. They – and, therefore, if they are employees, their employers – are liable only if they fail to reach the appropriate standards of expertise. Since experts may differ as to the correct diagnosis or treatment, a doctor or nurse will escape liability if they can prove the support of a 'responsible body of medical opinion' for their decision: *Bolam v. Friern Hospital Management Committee*, 1957.[38] In a sense, of course, this means that the medical profession sets its own standards of negligence.

A leading case on medical negligence and vicarious liability is *Stokes v. GKN*, 1968.[39] The company employed an occupational health doctor. He knew from medical literature and from a recent death within the company that continual contact with ordinary machine oil created a risk of scrotal cancer. At the time this hazard was not generally understood. The doctor had to decide what should be done to warn employees of the danger, without at the same time alarming them unnecessarily. He thought that since the risk was very small it was not necessary to run an all-out safety campaign. Instead, he gave talks to union officials which were sometimes relayed by word of mouth when the officials were collecting union dues. He adopted, as the judge subsequently said, a policy of 'soothing rather than alerting'. A few years later, Mr Stokes, a tool setter, whose overalls were often saturated with machine oil, died of scrotal cancer. In his widow's claim the judge said that while the risk might have been small, the consequences were fatal, and so the doctor should have advised a far more vigorous and effective safety campaign. His failure to do so was a serious error of judgement amounting to negligence, for which his employers were held liable.

We might note in passing certain other observations of the judge in this case, showing a commendable understanding of the sometimes difficult and delicate role of the occupational health practitioner.

A factory doctor when advising his employees on questions

of safety precautions is subject to pressures and has to give weight to considerations which do not apply as between a doctor and his patient, and is expected to give, and in this case regularly gave, to his employers advice based partly on medical and partly on economic and administrative considerations. For instance he may consider some precaution medically desirable but hesitate to recommend expanding his department to cope with it, having been refused such an expansion before; or there may be questions of frightening workers off the job or interfering with production . . . A factory doctor must use his own judgement and it must of course be recognized that he has pressures and considerations that weigh upon him; but that does not mean that he or those vicariously responsible for him are to be exonerated if he makes decisions, however honest, that he should have realized were wrong.

Course of employment

The second thing the plaintiff in a vicarious liability case must prove is that the employee's wrongful act was committed in the course of his or her employment. This is not decided simply by asking when or where the accident occurred. The question is essentially whether the action which caused the injury was **a way** of doing what the employee was supposed to do, even though it might have been a dangerous, stupid, careless or disobedient way of doing the job. That in turn means the employee may still be in the course of his/her employment despite the fact that he/she is acting in breach of his/her contract of employment: *Century Insurance v. Northern Ireland Road Transport Board,* 1942,[40] – employee unloading petrol while in breach of no smoking order – employer liable to pay for the damage.

The working of the rule is very clearly illustrated in *Iqbal v. London Transport*, 1973.[41] Here a bus conductor was waiting at the depot for his driver to come and turn the bus round, ready to begin the journey. In the driver's continued absence the conductor got in the cab and turned the bus round. As he did so he ran over a fellow employee, the plaintiff. The plaintiff claimed against the employer, on the basis that the conductor was on works premises, in works hours and acting – as he saw it – in the interests of the employer. But the court held nonetheless that the conductor was not in the course of his employment, since driving was not **a way**, even a disobedient way, of conducting. It was outside his employment altogether. The results of such a decision are very unfortunate for the injured person. He has sued the wrong party, and so is liable both for his own and the other side's costs. His only claim is against the wrongdoer, who probably has little or no money to meet the claim. In the end both wrongdoer and plaintiff may be bankrupted.

As a general rule, accidents caused by an employee's negligence when on his/her way to or from work, but not yet on site, are not in the course of his employment, whether or not he/she is paid for travelling time. Time and place and means of transport are all matters for the employee to decide. But if the employer authorizes or requires or controls a particular journey, he/she may thereby become responsible: *Smith v. Stages*, 1989.[42] Similarly, other activities of the employee which are merely **permitted** rather than required by the employer, and which are perhaps only for the employee's own benefit, are not likely to result in vicarious liability. This was the decision in the difficult case of *Crook v. Derbyshire Stone*, 1956,[43] where the employer escaped liability for an accident caused by his driver during a permitted rest break.

A final but important consideration is that, with rare exceptions, vicarious liability occurs only in the employer-employee relationship. On principle, an employer is not vicariously liable for the acts of independent contractors. Thus where an employer brings self-employed workers or another employer's employees on to his/her site for construction work he/she is not vicariously liable for their negligence.

STATUTORY PROTECTION

Health and Safety at Work Act

We have now considered the general principles of employers' liability at common law, breach of which entitles the injured person to claim damages. It remains only to say a little more about the protection given to people at work by Act of Parliament, and in particular by the Health and Safety at Work Act 1974. We have mentioned already some of the most important and recent regulations made under that Act, but there are several other provisions we should note.

The Act was based on the recommendations of the Robens Report of 1972 – a Royal Commission inquiry into industrial safety.[44] One of the report's main findings was that many accidents occurred because of employees' apparent indifference to their own safety. Employees seemed to think that accidents happened only to other people and that responsibility for safety was not their concern but that of the factories' inspectors. The report also criticized the complexity of industrial safety law and the resulting limitations on the powers of inspectors to take prompt, remedial action. Even when prosecutions were successful, magistrates often imposed derisory fines.

To overcome the first problem, that of apathy, the Act entitled employees (limited by Labour government reform to members of recognized unions) to appoint safety representatives at their places of work – a system previously adopted only in mines and quarries. Representatives must be given the facilities and assistance they may reasonably require and be consulted by the employer on all matters of safety, with a view to effective co-operation. They are entitled to paid time off for their work. They may require management to establish a safety committee with managerial participation. The committee can study the circumstances of accidents, conduct inspections, propose safety measures, and advise on safety education and compliance with safety rules. Further details, including provisions as to the training and numbers of representatives, are given in the Safety Representatives and Safety Committee Regulations 1977, as amended by the Management of Health and Safety at Work Regulations 1992.

As regards the overall complexity of the law and the limited powers of inspectors to enforce it, the Act made radical reforms. Instead of dealing with hazards on a piecemeal basis, as under previous legislation, the Act introduced a general duty on all employers to ensure so far as reasonably practicable the safety, health and welfare of their employees. This general duty, in effect a criminalized version of the common-law duty to take reasonable care which we have examined above, brought millions of workers under the protective umbrella of the criminal law for the first time. As we said at the beginning of this chapter, however, the law did not thereby impose any new safety duties upon employers; it merely added the possible penalties of the criminal law to existing civil obligations. Similar duties are imposed by the Act for the benefit of visiting contractors and others who may be affected by the employer's operations. Employees and the self-employed must obey safety rules, or may themselves be prosecuted.

The Act enables the Secretary of State for Employment to make regulations applying these general duties to specific issues. Apart from the regulations mentioned earlier, we should note the obligations imposed on employers under the Reporting of Injuries, Diseases and Dangerous Occurrences Regulations ('RIDDOR') 1985 to report to the Executive accidents causing more than three days' absence from work, certain work-related diseases or other mishaps, and a wide range of occurrences such as fires and explosions, whether or not they cause injury. All injuries must be recorded in an accident book. The Health and Safety (First Aid) Regulations 1981 prescribe the numbers and contents of first-aid boxes and lay down general principles on first-aid training. Recent regulations on particular hazards include those on lead, 1980; electricity, 1989; diving operations, 1991–92, and control of substances hazardous to health ('COSHH'), 1988.

Factories Act

The Factories Act of 1961 was the last of a long line of such Acts going back to the first ineffectual attempts at the beginning of the nineteenth century to protect workers against injury and exploitation. Much of the Act has now been repealed and replaced by regulations made under the Health and Safety at Work Act, but several important sections are still in force. A point of interest is that some of these sections impose strict liability, i.e., liability which, unlike that at common law or under the 1974 Act, does not depend on proof of fault. Under sections 22–7, for instance, all hoists, lifts, chains, ropes, lifting tackle and cranes must be soundly constructed, of adequate strength and properly maintained. The courts have decided accordingly that if a lift causes an accident, that can only be because it was not properly constructed or maintained – regardless of any evidence the employer might give as to regular inspection and servicing.

CONCLUSION

There is no doubt that the overall direction of the criminal law on health and safety at work is towards both simplification and greater effectiveness – subject, of course, to the appointment of sufficient numbers of inspectors. Prohibition and improvement notices are speedy and efficient remedies. In the courts, much higher fines are now imposed than would have been contemplated 10 or 20 years ago. To the extent that the criminal law works, it should help gradually to instil a general awareness of the importance of health and safety at work and eventually to reduce the accident rate.

But progress in that direction achieves nothing for those already injured and in desperate need of support. We have seen that claims for compensation generally depend on proof of fault. We have also seen that such claims are extremely expensive, long drawn-out and quite unpredictable in their outcome. Many people's claims end in failure and ruin, regardless of the extent of their injuries or needs.

We end therefore with a proposal for reform: that Britain should adopt an accident compensation scheme like the one introduced in New Zealand in 1974. The very short effect of this scheme is that all claims for damages for personal injury caused by accident are abolished. In their place is a rational and more or less comprehensive insurance scheme, whose operation depends on proof of **need** rather than **fault**. The basic rule is that anyone who can prove they have suffered injury by accident, however caused, resulting in loss of earning capacity, is entitled after two weeks to a weekly payment of 80% of that lost capacity, up to a maximum of approximately £350 a week. There are other assorted benefits including hospital treatment.

The New Zealand scheme is not perfect, of course, and its scope has been reduced by recent changes in the law. But it is still far more economical and efficient than litigation. Only some 6% of the total moneys involved in the New Zealand scheme goes on administration, whereas in Britain, for every £100 paid out in damages, approximately another £120 is spent on legal and insurance costs – and in the end, as we have said, many people get nothing. The New Zealand system recognizes that fault is the concern of the criminal law and that guilt or innocence should not be worked out at the expense of the injured party, as it is in Britain. The system actively fosters rehabilitation and accident prevention, contrary to that in Britain. It is a remarkably enlightened and humanitarian reform. Shall we ever see the like in Britain?

CASE REFERENCES

Cases noted in the text discuss in detail the issues raised there. The appropriate law report references are given in the footnotes below. The following list of law report abbreviations may be helpful for further reference:

AC:	Appeal Cases
All ER:	All England Reports
CLYB:	Current Law Year Book
ICR:	Industrial Cases Reports
IRLR:	Industrial Relations Law Reports
KIR:	Knights Industrial Reports
MedLR:	Medical Law Reports
PIQR:	Personal Injuries and Quantum Reports
SLT:	Scots Law Times
SolJ:	Solicitors' Journal
WLR:	Weekly Law Reports

NOTES

1. Figures from the Health and Safety Commission Annual Report 1991–2, which should be compared with those recorded in the Robens Report on Safety and Health at Work 1970–72, Cmnd. 5034.
2. Employers' Liability (Compulsory Insurance) Act 1969.
3. Dismissal on grounds of ill health is essentially a managerial rather than a medical issue: *Rolls Royce v. Walpole* [1980] IRLR 343 (Employment Appeal Tribunal).
4. [1953] AC 643.
5. (1989) *The Times*, 13 June.
6. [1977] SLT 66.
7. [1992] PIQR 57.
8. [1952] 96 SolJ852.
9. [1953] AC 180.
10. [1959] 1 All ER 81.
11. [1987] 3 WLR 212.
12. [1992] IRLR 34.
13. (1992) *The Times*, 29 Dec.
14. (1992) *The Times*, 2 July.
15. [1992] 3 Med LR 129.
16. [1990] IRLR 516.
17. [1991] IRLR 463.
18. (1972) 13 KIR 275.
19. [1992] IRLQ 349.
20. (1972) 13 KIR 255.
21. (1960) *The Times*, 22 Nov.

22. [1957] 2 All ER 229.
23. (1967) 3 KIR 28.
24. (1962) *Guardian*, 11 Oct.
25. (1961) 105 SolJ912.
26. [1990] ICR 61.
27. (1975) *The Times*, 25 Nov.
28. (1982) *The Times*, 29 Oct.
29. (1980) *The Times*, 19 July.
30. [1992] CLYB.
31. [1951] AC 367.
32. [1953] 2 All ER 391.
33. [1955] 2 All ER 12.
34. [1959] AC 743.
35. (1971) 12 KIR 13.
36. [1990] IRLR 516.
37. [1951] SLT 395.
38. [1957] 2 All ER 18.
39. (1968) 5 KIR 401.
40. [1942] AC 509.
41. (1973) *The Times*, 7 June.
42. [1989] IRLR 177.
43. [1956] 2 All ER 447.
44. Cmnd. 5034.

FURTHER READING

Encyclopedia of Health and Safety at Work (ed.) M. Goodman, Sweet and
    Maxwell, London.
Munkman, J. (1990) *Employers' Liability*, Butterworth, London.
Selwyn, N. (1993) *Law of Health and Safety at Work*, Butter-
    worth, London.
Stapleton, J. (1986) *Disease and the Compensation Debate*, Clarendon Press,
    Oxford.
Whincup, M. (1991) *Modern Employment Law*, Heinemann, Oxford.

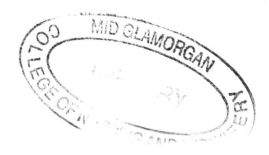

Index

Page numbers appearing in **bold** refer to figures, page numbers appearing in *italic* refer to tables